VAGUS NERVE SECRETS

How to activate your Vagus Nerve and how Access Your Body's Self-healing Power! Exercises to Activate Your Nervous System Stimulation, Overcoming Anxiety, Depression and trauma

By Roberta Rivera

Table of Contents

Introduction 1

Chapter 1 A Complete View Of The Nervous System 3

Chapter 2 The Vagus Nerve In Medical Therapy 25

Chapter 3 Central Cranial Nervousness (Mystery) 41

Chapter 4 Vagus Nerve Dysfunctional Signal 55

Chapter 5 How To Know If Your Vagus Nerve Is Injured Or Compressed 71

Chapter 6 Vagal Tone 78

Chapter 7 Health And Life Benefits 88

Chapter 8 Vagus Nerve: Its Importance To Weight Loss And Health 107

Chapter 9 Vagus Nerve Stimulation Techniques 114

Chapter 10 Stimulation Of The Vagus Nerve And Keeping It Healthy 136

Chapter 11 Vagus Nerve For Reducing Inflammation ... 152

Conclusion 174

Introduction

Vagus Nerve is a book that has been outlined in a professional manner, helping you understand all the physiological and social benefits of the nerve in simple terms. Although the Vagus Nerve is a complex anatomical part of your body, the language used in this book is simplified for all to understand. You do not have to be a doctor or conversant with medical terms in order to capture the concepts of the book. All the content is simplified to accommodate those who have a high degree of understanding and those who may not be very conversant with English.

Vagus Nerve is focused on outlining the importance of the nerve to your life. The book also helps you understand the procedure of caring for your Vagus Nerve. As we will observe throughout the book, the Vagus Nerve is a central part of your body functions. It is an integral part of your thinking and reaction. It influences your motion and emotions directly and must be protected from damage.

This book also helps you learn how to stimulate and activate the nerve. If the vagus nerve gets damaged or dysfunctional for one reason or another, you must be able to spot the symptoms and act upon them. This is only possible if you understand how the nerve can be activated. This book will help you find answers to important questions. You will learn how to cater to your vagus nerve's health as well as cater to the nerve when it is damaged.

There are natural ways of catering for your nerve. This book seeks to help you answer some vital questions while at the same time providing solutions to some problems. What can you do to ensure that your nerve remains functional? What are the foods that will stimulate your nerves? These are among the few questions that we will be answering.

Most importantly, this book seeks to give you a practical approach to dealing with some lifestyle and social conditions, including high blood pressure, anxiety, and depression. The vagus nerve is an integral part of your body that will help you calm down your tension and control diseases such as anxiety. Once you know how to stimulate and relax your nerve, you will be in a position to control impulsive conditions or any condition that is associated with emotional triggers.

Chapter 1 A Complete View Of The Nervous System

What Is The Nervous System In Detail?

The human body is made up of a complex system with multiple components that interact with each other. This complex system has a unique and difficult model for understanding due to dependencies, competitions, relationships, among other internal interactions within and without the system. This system can be compared to the nervous system; a part of the human body compromising of a network of nerve cells and fibers used as a channel for transmitting nerve impulses between body parts and to the Central nervous system which sends back information to the peripheral nervous system after it processes the information. Generally, the nervous system has two different types that include; diffuse and centralized. Lower invertebrates such as Protozoa, Porifera, and Coelenterata operate using the diffuse nervous system since there is no brain, and the neurons are distributed through the body in a netlike pattern. The centralized system is found in higher invertebrates, usually larger in sizes, such as Molluscs, Arthropods, and vertebrates, a class where human beings belong to operate on the centralized system that plays a big role in collecting information to trigger a response. For human beings, the nervous system is divided into two parts, namely; the Central Nervous system, with more nerves, and the peripheral nervous system.

Central Nervous System

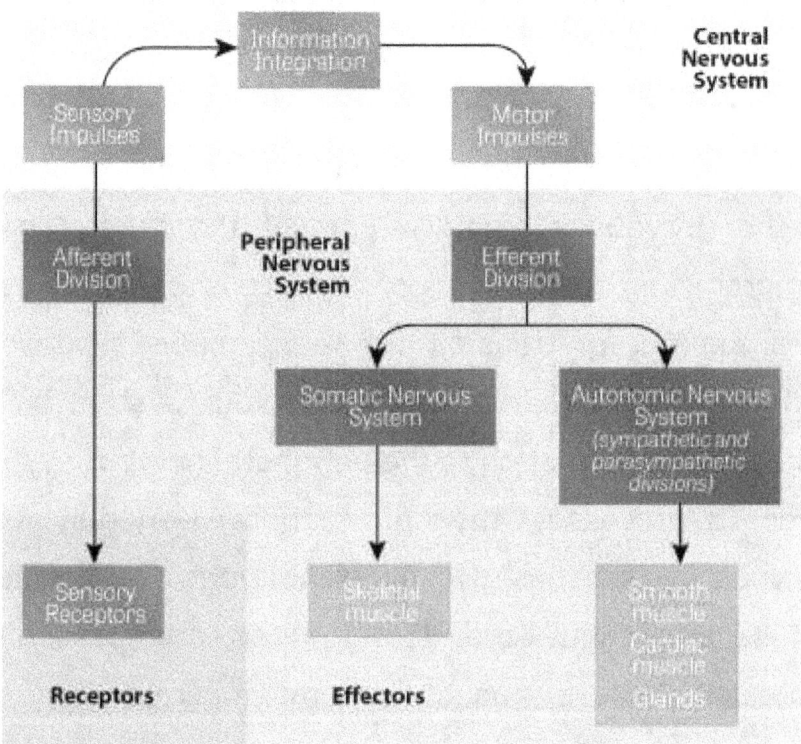

Central Nervous System

The central nervous system compromises of the brain and the spinal cord. The two organs integrate the information to influence any activity in the nervous system. The posterior surface of the human body hosts a dorsal body cavity that houses CNS while the cranial cavity and the spinal cavity houses the brain the spinal cord, respectively. The spinal cord and the brain lie along the posterior, and the cord is directly beneath the heart.

Peripheral Nervous System

This part of the nervous system consists of following distinct elements, namely nerves and ganglia, outside the brain and spinal cord. The peripheral nervous system connects the central nervous system forming a relay between the brain and spinal cord, including the limbs and organs. The system branches to the somatic nervous system, the autonomic nervous system, and the enteric system. Unlike the Central Nervous System, it is exposed to toxins for lack of protection from the vertebral column or even skull. The autonomous system is divided into parasympathetic and sympathetic systems. The SNS triggers muscle movement and is usually active to maintain a dynamic state of equilibrium, such as body temperature and body fluids. The system is an antagonist to the parasympathetic nervous system that activates the 'feed and breed' response and is most active when the body is inactive.

The parasympathetic system is also active when sexually aroused, salivating, crying, and when you are urinating. The enteric nervous system, which is also a useful part of the nervous system, operates independently, and it is responsible for continuous regulation of the gastrointestinal tract, a part of the digestive system.

The basic element in the nervous system is the nerve cell, also known as a neuron. These cells form the nerve and fibers. These nerves are protected by a fatty substance, also known as the myelin that acts as protection for the parts of fibers. The nervous system consists of both afferent nerves or sensory nerves. Both of these are responsible for taking information to a particular brain region as well as the efferent nerves and motor nerves responsible for taking out information from a specific region of the brain to trigger a response.

The nervous system is mandated with controlling body activity through basic units known as neurons. These are nerve cells distributed extensively in and out of body organs. Neurons in your body perform different activities; motor neurons, for example, are responsible for muscle movement; this is because they are tasked with transmitting messages from the brain to the muscles. Sensory neurons, on the other hand, assist you in recognizing light, noise, taste, smell, or even heat and in return, sending the information to the brain to trigger a response. Depending on the brain evaluation, you might close your eyes to protect yourself from the light, or you might simply start sweating to regulate body temperature in a hot environment. Interneurons are those nerve cells that connect various neurons within the brain and spinal cord.

Neurons compromise of the nerve cell body as well as extensions from the cell body known as dendrites and axon. Before the neurons receive any information, the dendrites collect and carry information to the designated cell body as the axons, and outward direction cell body takes the information from the cell. Information is then transmitted from neuron to neuron across the synapse, usually the gap separating these neurons.

The nervous system highly depends on an individual's genetics, and you will only have malfunctions of the system through genetic disorders, trauma, aging, physical damage, or intake of toxic substances. In the case of the system's malfunction, the peripheral nervous system is prone since due to its placement in the body that exposes it to toxins and bodily harm. The most common and noticeable defect mostly observed is the failure of this particular nerve to conduct stimuli that causes multiple sclerosis, and in a severe state, it may cause amyotrophic lateral sclerosis. These disorders cause damage to insulating covers in nerve cells that transmit deterred information or death of the nerve that completely stops the transmission of information through the nerves to the brain or a particular region in the body.

Nerves in the system, also known as fibers because of the existence of both axons and neurons, are cylindrical in shape as they form a pattern from the brain and spinal cord where they emanate before branching to the rest of the body. Neurons, however, have cell bodies that exist in different parts of the Central Nervous System: peripheral ganglia, spinal cord, and the brain.

The vertebrate nervous system is divided into areas known as gray matter and white matter. Gray matter is only cray in preserved tissue and changes color in living tissue, and it contains a large proportion of neurons. White matter consists of insulated axons, and its color often depends on the myelin. The matter contains all nerves and is majorly found in the brain and spinal cord.

Your nervous system compromises a network of nerve cells, also known as neurons. The millions of neurons in the body assist in transmitting information to a particular region, either in the brain or spinal cord. These two organs act as main stations in the Central Nervous System (CNS) and host to these neurons that consist of fibers known as dendrites and axons. Information in the Central Nervous System is integrated by the sensory impulses and motor impulses.

The sensory impulses are responsible for passing information about stimuli from within the body organs and outside the body and to the Central Nervous System. Motor neurons, on the other hand, instruct muscles and glands found in body organs in order to achieve a response. Interneurons or association neurons are found in the Central nervous system and not in the peripheral nervous system.

The Basic Cell Of The Nervous System

The basic functional cell of the nervous system is called neuron that transmits impulses. There are three types of neurons, sensory neuron, motor-sensory, and interneurons. The sensory neurons bring the message to Central Nervous System while motor neurons carry the message from the Central Nervous system. Interneurons act as intermediaries between sensory and motor neurons. A neuron responds to a stimulus, which is a change in the environment that causes a response and converts it into an impulse. The stimulus has to be strong enough to start and impulse. Impulses continue in the same strength throughout the neuron in a self-propagation manner.

Central Nervous System

The Central nervous system consists of the Brain and spinal code.

Brain

Brain stem- medulla, pons, midbrain

Diencephalon

Cerebellum

Cerebrum

Spine – Spinal Cord

Impulses eventually reach the brain through the sensory neurons. The brain processes the incoming impulses and decides on the response. The brain is a wave of interconnected nerve fibers (axons and dendrites). Meninges is a membrane that protects the brain and spinal cord. Where the fluid called cerebrospinal fluid fills the space between the two inner membranes. It acts as a shock absorber, therefore, protecting the Central Nervous System.

Sensory Impulses

This is the polarization and depolarization through which fiber activity spreads. The sensory neurons within the nervous system convert external stimuli from the organism's environment into internal electrical impulses. To achieve muscle contraction, the neurons respond to tactile stimuli. The nerve cell is, therefore, the nerve cord when your body carries sensory stimuli to the brain. Dendrites are the cytoplasmic extensions of the nerve cell. Sensory neurons carry electrical signals from the sensory organs to the Central Nervous System (CNS). They are afferent neurons since they are responsible for taking information to the brain.

Motor Impulse

Through the motor neuron, a motor impulse is achieved. This is the nerve cell that that is responsible for channeling impulses from the brain or spinal cord to the muscle or gland of a particular body organ. The motor impulse occurs once the neuron carries efferent impulses to the effector in order to trigger a response.

Dendrites contribute to the motor impulse by carrying the impulse triggered by the sensory neuron.

Peripheral Nervous System

The peripheral part of the system consists of nerves and ganglia. Nerves formed in net-like form make up the most part of the system, and they flow from the Central Nervous System and the spinal cord to the peripheral part of the nervous system. This part then divides into afferent and efferent parts under the sensory and impulse division, respectively.

Afferent Division

This part of the nervous system is where nerve fibers that convey information to the brain exist. They receive the message from the sensory receptors spread all over your body. Afferent signals travel away from the stimulus. For example, when you touch a hot object, the nerve endings in your fingers send a message to the brain that the hot object is painful, and therefore there is an urgent need for a response.

Efferent Division

The efferent division, on the other hand, consists of neurons that are also called motor neurons. These neurons relay or carry information away from the brain via fibers to necessary muscles and designated glands to facilitate response. For example, walking under the sun triggers the sending of information from the brain through the motor impulse that triggers your sweat glands to release sweat to regulate body temperature.

Autonomic Nervous System

As part of the nervous system process, this division operates unconsciously regulating bodily functions like breathing, sweating, urination, sexual arousal, digestion, pupillary, and heart rate, among other body activities. It contains three parts in order to achieve these processes and activities.

Somatic Nervous System

This part of your nervous system consists of afferent nerves and efferent nerves, and they also include all non-sensory neurons connected with the skeletal muscles and skin. The system is associated with the voluntary control of body movement s through the skeletal muscles. Nerve signals emanate from the upper cell bodies within the posterior portion of the frontal lobe. Stimuli from this part of the body are then sent from the upper motor neurons and down the corticospinal tract where the white matter terminating on the lower motor neurons and interneurons in the spinal cord. The information is sent through the axon, and this is when the system enables you to move your limbs or any other skeletal muscles.

Receptors

This is the part of the nervous system that is responsible for reacting to physical stimuli in the environment, whether internally or externally. The process is completed or achieved once the sensory nerve at the rear end receives information and undertakes a process of generating and aligning nerve impulses that are then transmitted to the brain through the interconnected fibers for interception and perception.

Effectors

These are cells that respond to stimuli from the sensory receptors through neurons. Effector's nerves serve both skeletal, smooth and cardiac muscles as well as glands. They are responsible for coordination and control once the brain sends electrical impulses to the skeletal muscles through the spinal cord and nerves. Effectors restore optimum levels, such as temperature and glucose levels. The responses are usually muscle contractions or hormone release.

Conclusion

You communicate to the outside world with the help of the nervous system. Responses and reactions upon receiving stimuli internally or externally. The nervous system receives information from your senses, processes the information that is then acted upon to trigger a response. The brain alone has 100 billion neurons in it, making it a major part of the nervous system. The axon that is responsible for passing information around is about a meter long; hence, the quick response in times of danger or haste.

There are two significant of the nervous system, namely the central and the peripheral nervous systems. The brain and the spinal cord form the central nervous system (CNS), while everything else is categorized under the peripheral nervous system (PNS). The nervous system organizes the majority of the body's exercises. It not only maintains the body's ability to adapt to crisis circumstances but also controls the upkeep of typical capacities Movement nerves pass on information from the CNS to the muscles and the organs of the body. The motor elements of the nervous system utilize peripheral neurons conveying the stimuli from CNS to effectors. Effectors, which are found on the outside of the nervous system, incorporate muscles and organs whose activities are either controlled or changed by nerve impulses.

Below are some of the functions of the nervous system.

- Sensation

The principal significant role of the nervous system is a sensation—getting data about nature to pick up contribution about what's going on outside the body (or, in some cases, inside the body). The tangible elements of the nervous system register the nearness of a change from homeostasis or a specific occasion in the earth, known as a boost. The faculties we consider most are the "huge five": taste, smell, contact, sight, and hearing. The improvements for taste and smell are both concoction substances (atoms, mixes, particles, and so on.), touch is physical or mechanical upgrades that communicate with the skin, locate is light boosts. Hearing is the view of sound, which is a tangible improvement like a few parts of touch. There are, in reality, a higher number of faculties than solely those, yet that rundown speaks to the significant faculties. Those five are on the whole detects that get boosts from the outside world, and of which there is conscious recognition. Extra tactile improvements may be from the inner condition (inside the body, for example, the stretch of an organ divider or the centralization of specific particles in the blood.

- Response

The nervous system delivers a reaction based on the boosts apparent by physical structures. A conspicuous response would be the development of muscles, for example, pulling back a hand from a hot stove. However, there are more extensive employments of the term. The nervous system can cause the compression of each of the three kinds of muscle tissue. For instance, skeletal muscle agreements to move the skeleton, cardiovascular muscle is affected as pulse expands during activity, and smooth muscle contracts as the stomach related framework move nourishment along the stomach related tract. Reactions likewise incorporate the neural control of organs in the body also, for example, the creation and discharge of sweat by the merocrine glands and eccrine found in the skin too frequently regulate body temperature. Reactions can be separated into those that are deliberate or cognizant (compression of skeletal muscle) and those that are automatic (withdrawal of smooth muscles, the guideline of cardiovascular muscle, and enactment of organs). The physical nervous system characterizes intentional responses, and the autonomic nervous system controls automatic responses.

- Integration

Enhancements that are gotten by stable structures are imparted to the nervous system where that data is prepared. This is called a mix. Improvements are contrasted and, or coordinated with, other upgrades, recollections of past boosts, or the condition of an individual at a specific time. This prompts the particular reaction that will be created. Seeing a baseball pitched to a hitter won't consequently make the player swing. The direction of the ball and its speed should be considered. Perhaps the check is three balls and one strike, and the player needs to release this contribute by the expectation of getting a stroll to initially base. Or then again, perhaps the player's group is such a long way ahead, it is amusing to swing endlessly.

Controlling The Body

The nervous system can be separated into two , generally based on a pragmatic distinction in reactions.

The sensory nervous system (SNS) is answerable for cognizant recognition and intentional engine reactions. A deliberate motor reaction implies the withdrawal of skeletal muscle. However, those compressions are not always willful as in you need to need to perform them. Some substantial engine reactions are reflexes and regularly occur without a cognizant choice to perform them. By any chance, your companion hops out from behind a corner and shouts, "Boo!" you will be caught off guard, and you may react by either shouting or jumping back. You didn't choose to do that, and you might not have needed to give your companion motivation to giggle to your detriment; however, it is a reflex, including skeletal muscle compressions. Other engine reactions become programmed (at the end of the day, oblivious) as an individual learns engine abilities (alluded to as "propensity learning" or "procedural memory").

The autonomic nervous system (ANS) is liable for automatic control of the body, generally for homeostasis (guideline of the inward condition). Tangible contribution to autonomic capacities can be from tactile structures tuned to outer or inside ecological boosts. The engine yield reaches out to smooth and cardiovascular muscle just as glandular tissue. The job of the autonomic framework is to manage the organ frameworks of the body, which typically intends to control homeostasis. Sweat organs, for instance, are constrained by the autonomic framework. At the point when you are hot, perspiring helps chill your body off. That is a homeostatic system. Be that as it may, when you are anxious, you may begin sweating moreover. That isn't homeostatic; it is the physiological reaction to an enthusiastic state.

There is another division of the nervous system that depicts practical reactions. The enteric nervous system (ENS) is liable for controlling the smooth muscle and glandular tissue in your stomach related framework. It is an enormous piece of the PNS and isn't reliant on the CNS. It is now and again legitimate, notwithstanding, to believe the enteric framework to be a piece of the autonomic framework because the neural structures that make up the enteric framework are a segment of the autonomic yield that directs absorption. There are a few contrasts between the two.

How Does The Nervous System Develop?

The development of the nervous system begins during prenatal development and later continues to develop after birth. As an embryo, the nervous system is developed through the birth and differentiation from the stem cell precursors, migration of immature neurons from their birthplaces in the embryo to final positions in the body. The process of growth in an embryo also involves the outgrowth of axons from neurons and guidance of the motile growth cone through the embryo towards postsynaptic partners that is then followed by the generation of synapses between the axons which assist in sending signals to particular parts of the body. In the adolescence stage of life, synaptic pruning involves decaying and dying off of both axon and dendrite as part of the synapse elimination process that begins in early childhood. Synapses later in life depend on learning and memory.

The development of the nervous system is divided into activity-independent mechanisms and activity-depended mechanisms. Activity-Independent mechanisms depend on your genetic program, usually played out in the neurons. It is a hardwired process, and they include; Differentiation, migration, and axon guidance to their prominent positions.

Neural Induction

During this process, the developing embryo's cells get transformed into unique and specialized tissue, which later develops into the spinal cord and brain. Mesoderm releases peptides to allow complete specialization of the cells. It begins with the neural plate that is usually at the top part of the embryo, which finally forms into a neural tube that flows from the brain to the rest of the body. Still, at the embryonic stage, the anterior part fully develops, forming the brain. The posterior part also develops to form the spinal cord.

Migration

Once the reproduction and division of cells have taken place, neurons attach to radial glial cells, and specialized glial cells climb along 'traveling' to their destination. The glial cells assume the responsibility of a guide to the neurons to their destination. Both active and passive cell migration is involved at this stage.

Passive Migration; The movement of the neurons formed first in the ventricular zone ends up at the top of the marginal zone. Neurons formed first have to be pushed by the cells growing underneath them.

Active Migration; During this process, the cells formed last are the ones that end up nearest to the marginal zone.

Migration occurs in the transition phase where the neuron becomes attached to the glial cell, the locomotory phase where the neurons move at the rate of 100 micrometers per day, and the recognition phase where the neurons recognize their destination and stop migrating.

Proliferation

Once the tube is fully closed, and you have the brain, cerebrospinal fluid forms in several layers to cushion the brain. This process is then followed by the formation of the forebrain, midbrain, and hindbrain that all play crucial roles when it comes to the operation of the nervous system. The four stages of cell division and multiplication occur in gradual growth to continue with neurogenesis, the production of nerve cells. Some of the cells already in the neural tube lose their capacity and begin to divide and reproduce. Neurons, however, do not divide since they are responsible for carrying electrical impulses with assistance from the glial cells that divide and reproduce at this stage.

Synaptogenesis

This is where cells connect with one another, forming the pattern of those connections. The growth cones found in axons and dendrites helps these cells find their target destination. This is done through long-distance zeroing in on an area and finding local addresses within that area.

Differentiation

This is the process where the cell changes from one type to another, and it occurs several times during development. This involves the growth of axons and dendrites, and this is when the adoption of a way of communication with other cells happens. Most neurons are formed maturely highly depending on the environmental influences that modify their form. Cell to cell interaction happens during this process, bypassing electrical signals to each other. Cell to cell communication is decided at this point depending on the individual since some neurons are totally connected without discontinuity, while some neurons have gaps between them while sending signals.

Chapter 2 The Vagus Nerve In Medical Therapy

Since the vagus nerve has such a large number of significant capacities, medicinal science has been keen on decades in utilizing vagus nerve incitement, or vagus nerve obstructing, in restorative treatment.

For a considerable length of time, the vagotomy system (cutting the vagus nerve) was a backbone of treatment for peptic ulcer malady, since this was a method for diminishing the measure of peptic corrosive being delivered by the stomach. Notwithstanding, the vagotomy had a few unfriendly impacts.

Today, there is extraordinary enthusiasm for utilizing electronic triggers (basically, changed pacemakers) to constantly invigorate the vagus nerve trying to treat different therapeutic issues. Such gadgets (alluded to conventionally as vagus nerve invigorating gadgets, or VNS gadgets) have been utilized effectively to treat individuals with extreme epilepsy that is headstrong to sedate treatment. VNS treatment is likewise now and then used to treat unmanageable misery.

Since when you have a sledge everything resembles a nail, organizations that make VNS gadgets are researching their utilization in a few different conditions including hypertension, headaches, tinnitus, fibromyalgia, and weight reduction.

Approaches to Unlock the Powers of the Vagus Nerve

The vagus nerve is the most significant nerve you presumably didn't have any acquaintance with you had.

In contrast to different Vegas, what occurs in this vagus doesn't remain there. The vagus nerve is a long wandering heap of engine and tactile strands that connections the mind stem to the heart, lungs, and gut. It additionally branches out to contact and cooperate with the liver, spleen, gallbladder, ureter, female ripeness organs, neck, ears, tongue, and kidneys. It powers up our automatic operational hub—the parasympathetic sensory system—and controls oblivious body capacities, just as everything from keeping our pulse consistent and nourishment assimilation to breathing and perspiring. It likewise directs pulse and blood glucose balance, advances general kidney work, helps discharge bile and testosterone, animates the emission of spit, helps with controlling taste and discharging tears, and assumes a significant job in ripeness issues and climaxes in ladies.

The vagus nerve has filaments that innervate for all intents and purposes the majority of our inward organs. The administration and handling of feelings happens through the vagal nerve between the heart, mind and gut, which is the reason we have a solid gut response to exceptional mental and enthusiastic states.

Vagus nerve brokenness can bring about an entire host of issues including weight, bradycardia (anomalous moderate heartbeat), trouble gulping, gastrointestinal ailments, swooning, mind-set issue, B12 lack, interminable aggravation, hindered hack, and seizures.

This Super Nerve (A Closer Look)

Be aware that just the spinal segment is a bigger nerve framework. Around 80 percent of its nerve strands—or four of its five 'paths'— drive data from the body to the cerebrum. Its fifth path keeps running the other way, moving sign from the cerebrum all through the body. Tied down in the cerebrum stem, the vagus goes through the neck and into the chest, parting into the left vagus and the correct vagus. Every one of these streets is made out of countless nerve filaments that branch into the heart, lungs, stomach, pancreas and about each other organ in the belly.

The vagus nerve utilizes the synapse acetylcholine, which animates muscle compressions in the parasympathetic sensory system. A synapse is a sort of synthetic dispatcher discharged toward the finish of a nerve fiber, that takes into account sign to be moved along from point to point, which animate different organs. For instance, if our mind couldn't speak with our stomach through the arrival of acetylcholine from the vagus nerve, at that point we would quit relaxing.

A few substances, for example, botox and the overwhelming metal mercury can meddle with acetylcholine creation. Botox has been known to close down the vagus nerve, which causes demise. Mercury obstructs the activity of acetylcholine. At the point when mercury appends to the thiol protein in the heart muscle receptors, the heart muscle can't get the vagus nerve electrical motivation for withdrawal. Cardiovascular issues typically pursue. Mercury utilized in fillings just crawls from the cerebrum just as the 3,000 tons of mercury put into the air can meddle with acetylcholine creation. Mercury-loaded immunizations may likewise assume a job in vagus nerve-related chemical imbalance in youngsters.

It's likewise accepted that diet assumes a job in vagus nerve wellbeing. An obesogenic 'cafeteria diet' (high-fat, high-carb lousy nourishment) decreases the affectability of the vagus nerve. Zesty nourishments can likewise make it fizzle.

This is on the grounds that the enteric sensory system (ENS), which oversees the capacity of the gastrointestinal tract, speaks with the focal sensory system (the mind) by means of the vagus nerve. This is known as the gut-cerebrum hub. The ENS is once in a while alluded to as the subsequent cerebrum or reinforcement mind focused in our sunlight based plexus.

The vagus nerve has strands that innervate for all intents and purposes the majority of our inside organs. The administration and handling of feelings happens by means of the vagal nerve between the heart, cerebrum and gut, which is the reason we have a solid gut response to exceptional mental and enthusiastic states.

Enthusiastic processing Emotional handling happens by means of the vagal nerve between the heart, mind and gut.

Vagus nerve brokenness can bring about an entire host of issues including stoutness, bradycardia (strangely moderate heartbeat), trouble gulping, gastrointestinal maladies, swooning, mind-set issue, B12 inadequacy, incessant irritation, disabled hack, and seizures.

The vagus nerve utilizes the synapse acetylcholine, which animates muscle compressions in the parasympathetic sensory system. A synapse is a sort of concoction errand person discharged toward the finish of a nerve fiber, that takes into account sign to be moved along from point to point, which invigorate different organs. For instance, if our cerebrum couldn't speak with our stomach by means of the arrival of acetylcholine from the vagus nerve, at that point we would quit relaxing.

Longest cranial nerve. The vagus nerve is the longest of our 12 cranial nerves.

A few substances, for example, botox and the substantial metal mercury can meddle with acetylcholine generation. Botox has been known to close down the vagus nerve, which causes demise. Mercury hinders the activity of acetylcholine. At the point when mercury appends to the thiol protein in the heart muscle receptors, the heart muscle can't get the vagus nerve electrical motivation for withdrawal. Cardiovascular issues typically pursue. Mercury utilized in fillings just creeps from the mind just as the 3,000 tons of mercury put into the climate can meddle with acetylcholine creation. Mercury-loaded antibodies may likewise assume a job in vagus nerve-related mental imbalance in youngsters.

The vagus nerve is consistently having an effect on everything in individuals with gut issues, nourishment sensitivities, weakness, nervousness, depersonalization, and cerebrum mist.

This implies individuals have an ease off vagal volume, i.e., having a lower capacity to play out its capacities.

The one issue to address in this circumstance is to discover which part of the vagus nerve is failing and to what degree it is the issue contrasted with different parts of your science.

Vagus nerve harm can likewise be brought about by diabetes, liquor addiction, upper respiratory viral contaminations, or having some portion of the nerve cut off inadvertently during an activity. Stress can arouse the nerve, alongside exhaustion and uneasiness. In any event, something as basic as awful stance can contrarily affect the vagus nerve.

The effect of stress can aggravate the vagus nerve, alongside weariness and nervousness.

It's additionally accepted that diet assumes a job in vagus nerve wellbeing. An obesogenic 'cafeteria diet' (high-fat, high-carb low quality nourishment) decreases the affectability of the vagus nerve. Fiery nourishments can likewise make it fizzle.

A Feeling in Your Gut

At the point when individuals state they feel it in their gut, that is not only creative mind, as indicated by Dr. Imprint Sircus, acupuncturist, and specialist of Oriental and peaceful medication.

Our gut impulses are not dreams however genuine apprehensive sign that guide quite a bit of our lives.

This is on the grounds that the enteric sensory system (ENS), which oversees the capacity of the gastrointestinal tract, speaks with the focal sensory system (the mind) by means of the vagus nerve. This is known as the gut-cerebrum hub. The ENS is now and then alluded to as the subsequent mind or reinforcement cerebrum focused in our sun based plexus. Sircus proceeds:

We presently realize that the ENS isn't only fit for self-governance yet in addition impacts the cerebrum. Truth be told, around 90 percent of the sign going along the vagus nerve come not from above, yet from the ENS.

Keeping the gut and vagus nerve passage solid effects our psychological wellness. An ongoing report demonstrates how anti-toxins can make us forceful when they upset the microbiome balance in our gut. A significant examination a year ago by McMaster University in Hamilton, Ontario, Canada, found that specific advantageous gut microorganisms can really counteract PTSD. However, probiotics can help keep vagus nerve flag and the gut in a more beneficial state, as indicated by a report in the National Center for Biotechnology Information (NCBI).

Vns Reduces Arthritic Inflammation Dramatically

A joint group of scientists from the United States and Amsterdam led a clinical preliminary inferred that by invigorating the vagus nerve with a little embedded gadget decreased aggravation essentially and improved results for patients with rheumatoid joint inflammation by hindering cytokine generation.

As per scientists, rheumatoid joint inflammation (RA) is a constant incendiary malady that has influenced over 1.3 million individuals in the United States and expenses more than a huge number of dollars to treat it every year.

For this examination, the neuroscientists and immunology-specialists utilized cutting edge innovation so as to delineate neural hardware that directs irritation.

One circuit, known as the "provocative reflex," there are activity possibilities that are transmitted in the vagus nerve which prevent the generation of cytokines.

This is viewed as the primary human investigation of its sort to diminish rheumatoid joint pain side effects by invigorating the vagus nerve with a little embedded gadget that set off a chain response and subsequently, decreased cytokine levels and aggravation.

What's more, despite the fact that the examination was centered around rheumatoid joint pain, the outcomes likewise gave constructive ramifications to individuals experiencing different infections, including Crohn's, Alzheimer's and Parkinson's.

Boosting With Electricity

Specialists have since quite a while ago abused the nerve's impact on the cerebrum. Electrical incitement of the vagus nerve, called vagus nerve incitement (VNS), is at times used to treat individuals with epilepsy or melancholy. VNS is intended to anticipate seizures by sending customary, gentle beats of electrical vitality to the cerebrum by means of the vagus nerve. These heartbeats are provided by a gadget something like a pacemaker. It is put under the skin on the chest divider and a wire keeps running from it to the vagus nerve in the neck. Scientists concentrating the impacts of vagus incitement on epilepsy saw that patients encountered a second advantage random to seizure decrease: their temperaments likewise improved.

According to a report distributed in the (PNAS) also known as Proceedings of the National Academy of Sciences (PNAS), indicated how invigorating the vagus nerve with a bioelectronic gadget "fundamentally improved proportions of infection action in patients with rheumatoid joint pain," a ceaseless provocative illness that influences 1.3 million individuals in the United States and costs several billions of dollars yearly to treat.

12 Vagus Nerve Stimulation Techniques

The vagus nerve shouldn't be stunned into shape. It can likewise be conditioned and reinforced like a muscle. Here are some basic things you can do that may improve your wellbeing especially:

1. Positive Social Relationships – An investigation had members contemplate others while quietly rehashing positive expressions about loved ones. Contrasted with the controls, the meditators demonstrated a general increment in positive feelings like tranquillity, happiness, and expectation in the wake of finishing the class. These positive musings of others prompted an improvement in vagal capacity as found in pulse changeability. The outcomes additionally demonstrated a more conditioned vagus nerve than when basically ruminating.

2. Cold – "Cold introduction, for example, chilly showers or face dunking invigorates the nerve also," says Mentore.

Studies demonstrate that when your body changes with cool, your battle or flight (thoughtful) framework decays and your rest and condensation (parasympathetic) framework increments and this is intervened by the vagus nerve. Any sort of intense cold introduction including drinking super cold water will build vagus nerve actuation.

3. Washing – Another home solution for an under-invigorated vagus nerve is to swish with water. Swishing really invigorates the muscles of the bed which are terminated by the vagus nerve.

"Ordinarily patients will tear up a piece which is a decent sign and and when they don't, we suggest that they do it consistently until they see that they do fire destroying a piece," says Hoffman. "This has been appeared to quickly improve working memory execution."

4. Singing And Chanting – Humming, mantra reciting, psalm singing, and playful enthusiastic singing all expansion pulse changeability (HRV) in marginally various ways. Basically, singing resembles starting a vagal siphon conveying loosening up waves. Singing as loud as possible works the muscles in the back of the throat to enact the vagus. Singing as one, which is regularly done in houses of worship and synagogues, likewise builds HRV and vagus work. Singing has been found to expand oxytocin, otherwise called the affection hormone since it makes individuals feel more like each other.

5. Back rub – You can invigorate your vagus nerve by rubbing your feet and your neck along the carotid sinus, situated along the carotid supply routes on either side of your neck. A neck back rub can help diminish seizures. A foot back rub help can bring down your pulse and circulatory strain. A weight back rub can likewise enact the vagus nerve. These back rubs are utilized to enable new-born children to put on weight by animating gut work, generally intervened by initiating the vagus nerve.

6. Chuckling – Happiness and giggling are common invulnerable sponsors. Giggling likewise animates the vagus nerve. Research demonstrates how chuckling expands HRV in a gathering domain.

There are different case reports of individuals blacking out from chuckling and this might be from the vagus nerve/parasympathetic framework being animated excessively. Swooning can come after giggling just as pee, hacking, gulping or solid discharge—which are all aided along by vagus initiation.

7. Yoga and Tai Chi — Both increment vagus nerve action and your parasympathetic framework when all is said in done. Studies have demonstrated that yoga expands GABA, a quieting synapse in your cerebrum. Scientists trust it does this by "invigorating vagal

afferents (strands)," which increment action in the parasympathetic sensory system. This is particularly useful for the individuals who battle with uneasiness or sadness.

Studies demonstrate that jujitsu likewise can 'upgrade vagal tweak.'

8. Breathing slowly and Deeply — Every human heart and the neck contains neurons that have receptors also known as baroreceptors, which identify circulatory strain and transmit the neuronal sign to your cerebrum. This enacts your vagus nerve that associates with your heart to lower circulatory strain and pulse. Slow breathing, with a generally equivalent measure of time taking in and out, expands the affectability of baroreceptors and vagal enactment. Breathing around 5-6 breaths for each moment in the normal grown-up can be extremely useful.

9. Exercise – Exercise expands your mind's development hormone, bolsters your cerebrum's mitochondria, and helps turn around psychological decrease. But at the same time it's been appeared to invigorate the vagus nerve, which prompts valuable cerebrum and emotional well-being impacts. Mellow exercise additionally

invigorates gut stream, which is interceded by the vagus nerve.

10. Espresso Enemas — Enemas resemble runs for your vagus nerve. Extending the entrail expands vagus nerve initiation, as is finished with douches. This purging is practiced by expanding the liver's ability to detoxify poisons in the blood and restricting them to the bile. All the while, the liver purges itself as it discharges the lethal bile into the little, at that point huge, digestive tract for clearing. The whole blood supply circles through the liver at regular intervals. By holding the espresso 12 to 15 minutes, the blood will circle four to multiple times for purging, much like a dialysis treatment. The water substance of the espresso invigorates intestinal peristalsis and purges the internal organ with the collected lethal bile.

11. Nervana — This wearable item sends a delicate electrical wave through the left ear waterway to animate the body's vagus nerve, while matching up with music, which thusly invigorates the arrival of synapses in the cerebrum that produce a quieting sensation all through the body.

12. Unwind – Learning how to chill might be the No. 1 thing to help keep your vagus nerve conditioned.

Chapter 3 Central Cranial Nervousness (Mystery)

The cranial nerve X is a vital part of the autonomic nervous system. Before Stephen Porges introduced Polyvagal theory, Vagus was thought to function as a single neural pathway. But we now know that the subspecies of the vagus nerve - ventral and dorsal - appear in different places and have very different functions, and this book is written to explain these differences and their implications.

The dorsal branch of the vagus nerve contains motor fibers that maintain the visceral organs under the respiratory membrane: the abdomen, liver, spleen, kidney, gall bladder, urinary bladder, small intestine, pancreas, ascending and transverse segments of the colon. Therefore, this branch is sometimes called the "membrane branch of the vagus nerve."

However, this description is only partially true, as some fibers originating from the dorsal motor heart of the brainstem also affect the heart and lungs above the membrane. Similarly, although the ventral vagus provides initial motor pathways of the organ above the membrane, some fibers affect the organs below the membrane.

The system - the dorsal and ventral branches of the vagus nerve, in the sympathetic chain of the spine - affect the vital functions of the respiratory and circulatory systems. Each of the three circles affects the heart and lungs in different ways.

The abdominal number of the vagus nerve is located in the brain stem, above the spinal cord below the brain. It stimulates the rhythmic narrowing of the bronchial, and facilitates oxygen extraction, while brain stimuli that control dorsal vaginal activation can lead to chronic narrowing of the airways, making it difficult to obtain air. (This is part of the mechanism that is activated in a state of circuits or trauma. Stenosis also occurs in chronic obstructive pulmonary disease, chronic bronchitis, and asthma.) If we feel safe, the ventral nerve of the vagus nerve supports rest or quiet activity. There is a rhythmic holiday to open the air passages. Moderate in power outages and moderate in an outbreak. Abdominal count of the vagus nerve inside many small muscles in the neck, including the vocal cords, larynx, pharynx, and some muscles around the back of the pharynx (Sling Philly Palatine and UV muscles).

A high cranial nerve, or "accessory nerve," is one of the keys to the well-being of the entire musculoskeletal system. Because it engages the trapezoid and sternocleidomastoid (SCM) muscles that allow head and neck movement, the tension in any of these muscles pulls on one side of the shoulder, spine, and the entire body.

Both the trapezoid as well as sternocleidomastoid muscles arise on the skull bones. (Trapezoid lends itself to the mastoid process of the temporal bone, the sternocleidomastoid cells of the occipital bone). Together they form the outer ring of the muscles of the neck, shoulders, and upper back.

If the high cranial nerve suffers from dysfunction, it leads to a deficiency of the right tone in these muscles. This, in turn, can cause acute or chronic shoulder problems, stiff neck, migraines, and face-to-face rotation.

Instead of just a trapezoid, loose massage, or SCM muscle, it is better for the therapist to first improve the function of the eleven cranial nerve with the basic exercise (see Part II), then the muscles. For massage, after the nerve works again.

Treatment Of Cranial Nerves

We need different techniques to treat cranial nerves than those commonly used to treat spinal nerves. For the treatment of spinal nerve weakness, some therapists use chiropractic or chiropractic fillings (short, high-speed expressions). A physical therapist can stretch and strengthen the muscles around the neck and return to the position of the spine, thereby reducing the pressure on the spinal nerves.

When these methods do not exist, we sometimes resort to orthopedics.

But if we want to improve or restore function manually in the cranial nerves, we need a different approach. Since 1920, there has been a form of treatment for the treatment of cranial neuropathies, called "cranial osteochondrosis" or "craniofacial therapy (CST)" or "cranial osteoarthritis (OCF)."

In the United States, orthopedic doctors receive the same training as doctors. Like its medical counterparts, she is licensed to perform surgeries, write prescriptions, and work in psychiatric hospitals. An important difference between orthopedists and medical muscles is that orthopedists have additional training and practical treatments.

William Garner Sutherland, DO (1873-1954) founded skull osteochondrosis. His student and colleague Harold Magon, DO (1927–2011), wrote the basic book "Osteoporosis in the Cornell Field," eight which was first published in 1951 and is still used today by orthopedic physicians who have chosen to learn skull techniques.

Mason's book describes three approaches to skull work. One is biomechanics, where the therapist holds two bones from the neighboring skull for the purpose of mobilizing them in the stitches (where two or more bones of the skull meet). This can reduce mechanical pressure on the cranial nerves as they pass through the various openings of the skull.

The biomechanical approach requires a detailed study of skull anatomy, as well as extensive practical experience of working sensing and using techniques effectively. French orthopedic surgeon Alain Gehen developed the biotechnology system as described by Sutherland and Magon, and taught his approach to students in many countries.

Another method of treatment in the skull includes dilation of soft tissue membranes within the skull and spine. The dura mater is a tube of connective tissue from the skull to the tail bone containing the brain, spinal cord, and cerebrospinal fluid.

All these parietal structures become less resilient with the aging, disease, certain types of antibiotics, and physical trauma. Harold Magon described these membranes and how tension in them could fade. Later, this work was developed by John Upledger, DO, and is now taught worldwide by the Upledger Institute in Florida. Its method involves extending wall membranes as well as "cooling" them.

The third approach is called craniofacial therapy. Its goal is to maximize the movement of cerebrospinal fluid that circulates around the brain and spine, introduce nutrition into substances and help eliminate metabolic waste products.

Biodynamic techniques facilitate the release by utilizing the flow of cerebrospinal fluid and parietal membranes of the skull and spine. The therapist grabs the client's head with a very light touch, along with a keen awareness of the small, delicate movements in the skull bones.

Spinal Nerves

Most people have heard about problems that arise from spinal dysfunction. Many people have a herniated hernia that presses the spine or bone growth (spinal stenosis) that can compress the spinal nerve and cause pain, loss of sensation, or functional loss (for example, bladder control). Spinal nerve dysfunction can also cause local paralysis (the inability to use specific skeletal muscles). Some people use chiropractic or orthopedic orthotics to relieve spinal nerve pressure. Chiropractors typically use high-speed and short-thrust techniques, designed to position the spine to make it better align and relieve pressure from the aching nerve. Orthopedists have the same goal but are usually gentler.

Other common "conservative" treatments for the spine are yoga and stretching, strengthening back muscles with calisthenics, weight training, physiotherapy, and massage to balance back tone muscles. If this method tries to maintain the shape of the spine, we may feel unhealthy, desperate, and tend to choose radical treatments such as surgery.

Back surgery is a thriving business. About 500,000 Americans undergo lumbar surgery each year. According to the US Agency for Research and Quality of Healthcare, in 2008, we spent more than $ 30.7 billion on hospital procedures to treat back pain. Studies show that most backpacks have gone through their time and effort. The hospital in the cities of Denmark and Denmark stopped using back pain surgery.

For decades, orthopedic surgeons have been treating back problems by cutting off part of the massive disc, cutting off the bone, or even inserting a metal plate and screws to reinforce adjacent vertebrae. Despite the extensive use of surgery, the effectiveness of these operations has not been scientifically documented. On the contrary, there is a growing body of research showing that such processes are not effective in the long run. 11, 12, 13

An important function of the spinal nerves is to allow us to use our arms, legs, and torso to move our bodies by relaxing and relaxing the various muscles. Spinal nerves excite some visceral organs. The messages originate in the spinal nerves in the brain and travel through the spine, a tear-like nerve hole that emerges from the skull through a large opening at the base of the skull called the foramen (Latin for "big hole").

Upon entering the skull, pairs of spinal nerves emerge from the spine, formed from a vacuum between adjacent vertebrae to serve the muscles, joints, ligaments, tendons, internal organs, and skin. Humanity has thirty-three pairs of spinal nerves, with one nerve from each pair on the right side of the body and the other on the left.

Each pair of spinal nerve corresponds to a portion of the spine. There are thirty-three vertebrae in total: seven in the neck, twelve in the chest, five in the lumbar region, five in the sacrum, and four in the tailbone. Spinal nerves, which contain both motor and motor nerves, carry back and forth signals between the brain and the rest of the body. Two important exceptions are:

Trapezoid and sternocleidomastoid muscles of the neck and shoulder, which receive their nerves from the elevated cranial nerve. There is always more than one branch of the spinal nerve in each particular muscle. This provides confirmation that if one of the spinal nerves is nervous, the muscles may still function (even less efficiently) by using signals from other available nerves.

All spinal nerve also affects different muscles. Muscles are often part of a series of motion - for example, the muscles of the shoulder, upper arm, forearm, wrist, and fingers act as a unit to control the basic movements of the arm or hand. The highways of the nerve indicate muscle contraction. Spinal sensory nerves collect different types of information from the body and feed them back to the brain: they carry pain sensations, the locations of the parts of the body relative to each other, movement, the tension in the muscles or fascia, and a sense of touch for the entire body except the face (transmitted through the cranial nerves). The branches of the spinal and cranial nerves are traditionally classified into the motor and sensory functions, but this is overly simplistic. If we look closely at individual "motor nerves," we notice that some of their fibers are motor fibers - but they also contain sensory fibers that report muscle tension to the brain. We now know that the majority of fibers in "motor nerves" are actually sensory.

This combination of sensory and motor nerve fibers provides a synthesis of reactions that allows us to use motor fibers to tighten muscles, while sensory fibers simultaneously send information to the brain about variable voltage levels in muscles. This allows us to calibrate muscle tension - a stronger and more effective approach than if the muscles cannot fully or completely tension, and this will be the case if we do not have sensory fibroblastic reactions.

Under normal conditions, spinal nerves facilitate easy and well-coordinated movements and burn muscles by reaching the minimum energy for the desired movement. However, when the body is in a state of tension, and all the muscles are too tight, this natural coordination often loses, and movements become uncoordinated, disturbed, or weak.

Spinal nerve branches are directed to specific physical structures: skin (skin tumors), muscles (myotomes), visceral organs (fillings), ligaments, fascia, and connective tissue (fascia atoms). Instead of an individual spinal nerve that has only one muscle, there is some overlap, so different spinal nerve branches can make the same individual muscles inside. This creates a backup system so that if one part of the nerve is damaged, the other parts can still move the same muscles, and can continue to work, even if it works less efficiently.

Some spinal nerves enter the internal organs. For example, nerves from the thoracic vertebrae T1 and T4 enter the heart, nerves from T5 and T8 go to the lungs, T9 goes to the abdomen, and T10 goes to the kidneys. Other nerves serve other structures, including the bladder, genitals, and intestines.

When the spine is ejected, some fibers of the thoracic spinal nerve and the upper part (T1 - L2) are extended horizontally for a short distance. While some are still in the same area, others step in and enter the vertebrae from the top and bottom to form part of the sympathetic chain. The sympathetic chain extends the length of the spine between T1 and L2, connected to these spinal nerves. Most sympathizers, who plan on the visceral organs and on the head, accompany the arteries to their destinations. When we pose a threat to our survival, there is a course of activity in the entire sympathetic chain that spreads the fight or flight response to mobilize the entire body's resources. This answer is direct and complete and is appropriate if we are threatened or threatened. Muscle tension to prepare for the movements necessary to fight or escape; this is described in weightlifting circles as "pumping."

Some organs within these friendly nerve fibers increase their activity levels to support this mobilization. For example, the heart beats faster to deliver more blood to the muscle system. Increases blood pressure to pump more blood into tight muscles. The liver frees sugars stored in the blood to provide additional energy to burn muscles. The survival stress response in the sympathetic chain causes the bronchial muscles to stop, improve our ability to breathe, and absorb the maximum amount of oxygen to mobilize or operate fully. At the same time, other organs are slowed or stopped (especially those involved indigestion). It is loss of appetite, slowing down or stopping the movement of food in the intestine, and may develop a sensation "Butterflies" in her stomach. In situations of threat or challenge, the state of stress resulting from the friendly response affects the entire body and may include muscles of all sectors at the same time. Activation of the cervical sympathetic chain and the "fight or flight" response is one of the three possible states of the autonomic nervous system, which will be later.

Intestinal Nervous System

The intestinal nervous system is a network of nerves connecting the visceral organs. We do not know anything about these nerves; because they are so closely related, with visceral organs and connective tissues between organs, it has so far been impossible for anatomists to follow the entire course of intestinal nerves. Therefore, we do not find them well represented in most anato.

Moreover, we know almost nothing about how complex nerves work. At best, we can advise that anatomical nerves somehow communicate with the various visceral organs to coordinate a highly complex digestive process.

The intestinal nervous system is also sometimes referred to as the "second brain," which has intelligence that works on our consciousness.

Chapter 4 Vagus Nerve Dysfunctional Signal

The vagus nerve may dysfunction when it is exposed to extremely stressful conditions. Sometimes, you may not be able to tell when the nerve is dysfunctional. Normally, the symptoms associated with vagus nerve dysfunction are also associated with other conditions. You may be fooled to think that you are suffering from a different infection, yet it is due to nerve damage. We have observed that the vagus nerve supports several activities and that all the activities are vital in your daily routine. A slight dysfunction of the nerve can put most of these activities to a halt or may affect the way you function.

There are two main causes of vagus nerve dysfunction: vagus nerve damage and vagus nerve inflammation. Vagus nerve damage is a much complex subject, and we will be looking at it in the following . At this level, all you have to note is that damage may lead to many health complications. The symptoms for vagus nerve damage may be very similar to the nerve stressing ones.

Vagus nerve stress can happen at any time or any day. As we delve deeper, we will be looking at environmental and social factors that can stress your vagus nerve. Knowing that the nerve can be stressed should raise the alarm on how you cater to your vagus nerve. It is necessary that you protect your nerve from any damage. All instances that may lead to the stressing of your vagus nerve must also be avoided.

Before we look at the symptoms of vagus nerve dysfunction, we should try and find out the possible ways of proving the dysfunction. As already mentioned, the symptoms for a dysfunctional vagus nerve are the same as those for a damaged nerve. The only way to be sure whether your nerve is dysfunctional or damaged is to undergo medical tests. There are several tests that can be used at a local health facility or even at home.

Doctors use the gag reflex test to determine the response of the nerve. In this test, a doctor will insert some soft tissue, maybe a cotton bud into your throat, and try to swab it on both sides. Normally, if the vagus nerve is functioning properly, the patient is supposed to feel a tickling sensation resulting in a gag. However, if the nerve has been damaged, the person may not feel anything. Other advanced tests can be used to determine the state of the vagus nerve, as we will see later on. There are different tests for diagnosing a damaged nerve, and there are individual tests that you can perform at home. However, this particular test is ideal for any individual who wishes to gain some certainty about the functioning of their vagus nerve. Before you jump into treating the nerve dysfunction, try to check the cause and make sure you have certainty that it is damaged.

Early Symptoms of Vagus Nerve Dysfunctional

There are clearly observable symptoms of vagus nerve dysfunction. However, some of these symptoms may be very diverse such that, most people never associate them with the vagus nerve. In most cases, the symptoms are associated with common conditions. If you realize that you are experiencing several of the following symptoms, it is wise to get a doctor's opinion on the health status of your vagus nerve.

- Difficulty Speaking or Loss of Voice: We have mentioned that laryngeal is the extension of the vagus nerve that extends directly to the voice box. This nerve is important in coordinating and controlling the activities of the voice box. If the nerve is damaged, muscle contraction and expansion becomes a complex duty. For this reason, any person suffering from vagus nerve damage or dysfunction is likely to suffer from voice problems.

- A Voice That Is Hoarse or Wheezy: This is still a part of the integral functions of the laryngeal. If you find out that your voice is getting horse or wheezy, the chances are that your vagus nerve has become dysfunctional. With that said, it is important to note that most people experience a wheezy voice during many instances. A simple cold could lead to a wheezy voice. This is the reason why it is important to get an opinion from the doctor before jumping into a conclusion about any symptom.

- Trouble Drinking Liquids: We have observed that the vagus nerve plays an important role by providing motor action to some parts of the body. The most integral parts of the body where the nerve plays such a role include the pharynx. The laryngeal extension of the vagus takes action on the pharynx and stylopharyngeus muscles that affect the swallowing of food. We have determined that the vagus nerve has an effect on the muscles that determine taste and also affects the production of certain enzymes. If you start realizing that you cannot swallow drinks, the chances are that your nerve is dysfunctional.

- Loss of the Gag Reflex: When you touch an object at the back roof of your mouth, the back muscles of the throat close automatically. This is what we refer to as the gag reflex. The gag reflex is very important since it helps a person swallow food and drinks. The reflex also plays an important role in separating the food pipe and the air pipe. In other words, if you did not have a gag reflex, the chances are that foods might find their way into the lungs. The fact that the vagus nerve controls your gag reflex means that any dysfunction of the nerve may lead to a lack of gag reflex. This option also provides one of the most reliable ways of testing your vagus nerve health. If you try touching the roof of your mouth close to the throat, you must experience an automatic closure of the throat muscles. This will give you a guarantee that your vagus nerve is still functional.

- Pain in the Ear: A branch of the vagus nerve known as auricular nerve extends to the ears. This nerve plays an important role in controlling the hearing of an individual. As a matter of fact, the auricular directly influences your sound senses. You may never be able to perceive sound well if the nerve is damaged. Pain in the ear is one of the obvious signs that the vagus nerve has been damaged. This is because the pain can only be caused by a fracture on the nerve.

- Unusual Heart Rate: The fact that the vagus nerve is linked to the heart means that any damage to the nerve may directly affect the heart rate. The cardiac extension of the vagus nerve determines the contraction of the heart muscles. This extension also helps in maintaining a steady flow of information between the heart and the brain. If the sensory nerves of the heart fail to function, the chances are that the heart may fail or may show abnormal rates. The normal heart rate is around 72 bits per second. In the case where the rate goes beyond 72, the patient should either be involved in cardiovascular exercises or the vagus nerve may be exposed to stress leading to the increased production of adrenalin.

- Abnormal Blood Pressure: We have established that the vagus nerve also affects the constriction of blood vessels. If the nerve is stimulated or under stress, it may lead to the constriction of blood vessels. Given that pressure may also lead to an increased heart rate, this simply means that over-stimulation of the nerve may cause increased blood pressure. When the heart is pumping at fast rates, yet the blood vessels have been constricted, the blood pressure is bound to increase. Such occurrences may lead to heart attacks or loss of consciousness. If you experience increased blood pressure constantly, you need to try and figure out the triggers. If your pressure is caused by vagus nerve stimulation or failure, the chances are that your nerve is malfunctioning. However, you should also remember that no all blood pressure issues are associated with the vagus nerve. Some of the blood pressure issues are associated with other lifestyle diseases.

- Decreased Production of Stomach Acid: We have also established that the vagus nerve works in conjunction with endocrine glands to ensure that food is digested. Before endocrine glands can produce the necessary enzymes that are needed in food digestion, they must receive signals from the autonomic nervous system. The most central part of the anatomic nervous system is the vagus nerve. If you realize that you are experiencing some of the symptoms of low stomach acids such as bloating, belching, heartburns, among others, you should start observing for other signs of vagus dysfunction. These symptoms may appear in short intervals if your vagus nerve is ailing. If the nerve is completely damaged, you may experience such conditions continuously.

- Nausea or Vomiting: Nausea and vomiting are also some of the symptoms that indicate high levels of stomach acid. If the vagus nerve is affected, it is possible to suffer from nausea and such symptoms. This is because the regulatory tissues that control the production of stomach acid are not functioning properly.

- Abdominal Bloating or Pain: The abdomen is the final destination of the vagus nerve, with the final ending touching the spinal cord. The fact that the nerve is extended to the lower abdomen means that if it is affected, you may experience some defects in your body. Given that the nerve plays an important role in controlling stomach muscles, it can be painful, leading to abdominal pain in some people.

Advanced Symptoms of Dysfunctional

The above symptoms are general and can apply to any person who has a dysfunctional vagus nerve. However, there are cases where the nerve is severely wounded or is completely damaged. In such cases, the symptoms tend to advance. In most cases., when the damage is, to a large extent, the focus is on diseases that may result from the vagus nerve damage.

In the above, we only focused on general symptoms that may relate to any problem to the nerve. However, as you advance to the next stages, you realize that the extent of damage to the nerve may cause some serious illnesses. There are two main diseases that doctors have linked to vagus nerve damage. We will look at these diseases in detail as we advance. In this , we only want to look at the symptoms and how they may be a way of showing that you have a dysfunctional vagus nerve. If you cannot detect or diagnose a defective vagus nerve, you may end up living in pain for a long time without being able to tell the cause. You may even be misdiagnosed by doctors if you do not know the right information about that condition. The two main conditions that may affect a person due to a damaged vagus nerve include gastroparesis and vasovagal syncope.

Gastroparesis

Several research findings have shown that there is a direct link between gastroparesis and vagus nerve damage. This is a condition that severely affects the involuntary contraction of the digestive system. As we had mentioned, the vagus nerve, in conjunction with ANS facilitates the parasympathetic functions of the body. Some of the parasympathetic functions include involuntary contraction of the digestive system. In simple terms, when you suffer from a damaged vagus nerve, you may never enjoy parasympathetic actions of defecation. The stomach does not empty properly, and this leads to a continuous pile up of dirt. Some of the common symptoms of this condition include

- Nausea or Vomiting: In the symptoms above, we mentioned nausea and vomiting. However, this case is much worse and severe. In the case of gastroparesis, the patient is unable to let out most of the food eaten. This leads to nausea and vomiting of foods long hours after eating. In normal vomiting situations, a person just vomits a few minutes after eating. However, in these advanced cases of gastroparesis, the victim is likely to vomit after very many hours of waiting.

- Loss of Appetite: Most people who suffer from gastroparesis, often eat a little food and constantly lack appetite. This condition makes a person feel full even when they are hungry. Patients suffering from this condition may either completely lack appetite or feel full after eating just a little amount. However, there are many other conditions that may still lead to a lack of appetite. Do not be quick to jump to conclusions just because a person lacks appetite. If you feel that you are suffering from a lack of appetite, investigate all the possible causes. You may also have a doctor test you for vagus nerve dysfunction.

- Acid Reflux: Acid refluxes will just occur as it is the case above. However, in this case, they will be much more severe and may be recurrent.

- Abdominal Pain or Bloating: The other direct symptom of gastroparesis is bloating and abdominal pain. The vagus nerve spreads to the lower abdomen, having an influence on your excretory and sexual organs. This means that any damage to the nerve may directly affect your sexual health or your digestive health. Such conditions will often lead to abdominal pain.

- Unexplained Weight Loss: There are several reasons why a person suffering from gastroparesis may lose weight. First, such individuals do not eat as much as they should eat. This means that the body is denied some of the essential vitamins. Further, the body does not fully digest the food consumed. In most cases, the food has to come out through vomit. Such issues often lead to a loss of weight in most patients — this a distinctive observation for the severe stage of vagus nerve damage. In the early symptoms, the patient may experience digestive complications, but they are not to the extent of affecting personal weight. In essence, those who suffer from the early stages of vagus nerve damage still have a choice to make on the types of foods they want to eat. They may still eat without vomiting. However, the stage where gastroparesis develops, it is almost impossible to manage the effects associated with eating.

-     Fluctuations in Blood Sugar: If you do not eat properly, you will end up affecting your blood sugar. The human body's blood sugar is balanced by the food being processed into glucose and absorbed into the system. However, if the stomach is not in a position to digest all the food that you eat, you are likely to encounter severe shortages in energy and blood sugar.

We have mentioned that some traditional treatment methods advocate for the removal of the vagus nerve through a process known as vagotomy. In this process, part of the nerve was cut off to help patients who suffer from increased stomach ulcers. However, it was realized that this process had several side effects. One of the most severe side effects associated with the vagotomy was the development of gastroparesis. It was realized that patients who underwent the process suffered advanced symptoms only associated with this condition.

Vasovagal Syncope

It is common for the vagus nerve to overreact to stress or stimulation. In the case of an overreaction, the vagus nerve may develop a condition known as vasovagal syncope. This condition can lead to a sudden drop in heart rate and blood pressure. If a person undergoes an extreme stressing situation that directly affects the vagus nerve, the drop in pressure may result in loss of consciousness (fainting). This is the condition that is known as vasovagal syncope. It is important to remember that the vagus nerve plays a central role in stimulating several muscles in the heart that directly affect your heart rate. If the nerve is overstressed, it may lead to a slowdown in the body processes leading to this condition.

Some of the extreme pressure events that can lead to vasovagal include:

- Exposure to Extreme Heat: Exposure to extreme heat all over sudden or for long hours may lead to excessive dilation of blood vessels. The dilation, in conjunction with the reduced pressure due to stress, may result in low blood pressure and a slow heart rate. This scenario is likely to lead to a loss of consciousness.

- Fear of Bodily Harm: Most people react differently to emotional situations. The emotion of fear has the strongest effect on the vagus nerve. When a person is afraid, excessive levels of adrenaline are produced to start the fight or flight state of the body. In this state, the vagus nerve is under extreme pressure. If someone was to startle you in the dark, you might undergo this type of excessive pressure. This may lead to a sudden drop in blood pressure and lead to a sudden loss of consciousness. In some people, the same action may lead to increased heart rate, increased blood pressure, and body heat. It is common to see people sweating under intense fear.

- The Sight of Blood or Having Blood Drawn: If you have fear for blood or if you fear needles, you may also undergo vasovagal syncope. This is common when a person sees blood for the first time. Since the picture blood creates a situation of intense fear, you are likely to stress the vagus nerve. This may lead to a sudden drop in blood pressure and heart rate, and as a result, lead to fainting.

- Straining: One of the ways to detect that a person is suffering from vasovagal is by observing the strain they go through. If you find yourself straining to have bowel movements, the chances are that you are suffering from vasovagal syncope. The pressure on the vagus nerve usually affects the digestive system and may lead to reduced intestinal action.

- Standing for a Long Time: Standing for a long time may create pressure on the vagus nerve. One of the reasons being that the upper body needs support to hold the nerve. When the neck and thorax muscles have to support themselves on the nerves for long hours, a person may experience problems in the natural flow of blood. This explains why it is common for people to faint after standing for long hours. The long hours may lead to a drop in heart rate and blood pressure and eventually lead to fainting.

Chapter 5 How To Know If Your Vagus Nerve Is Injured Or Compressed

Your fringe nerves are the connections between your cerebrum and spinal rope and the remainder of your body. Fringe nerves are delicate and effectively harmed.

Nerve damage can influence your cerebrum's capacity to speak with your muscles and organs. Harm to the fringe nerves is called fringe neuropathy.

Extending or pushing on a nerve can cause damage. The nerves additionally might be harmed because of other wellbeing conditions that influence the nerves, for example, diabetes or Guillain-Barre disorder.

In carpal passage disorder, weight on the middle nerve in the wrist causes harm. Or on the other hand the nerves might be squashed, cut or harmed in a mishap, for example, games damage or an auto collision.

Now and then in a fringe nerve damage, either the strands or the protection are harmed. These wounds are bound to recuperate.

In increasingly extreme fringe nerve wounds both the filaments and the protection are harmed, and the nerve might be totally cut. These kinds of wounds are exceptionally hard to treat and recuperation may not be conceivable.

For instance, perhaps you feel shivering or deadness or create shortcoming in your leg, arm, shoulder or hand, you may have harmed at least one nerves in a mishap. You may likewise encounter comparative side effects if a nerve is being packed because of elements, for example, a limited path, tumor or different sicknesses.

Serious fringe nerve wounds may make all out loss of inclination the zone where the nerve is harmed.

It's critical to get restorative consideration for a fringe nerve damage as quickly as time permits since nerve tissue now and then can be fixed. Early analysis and treatment now and again can avert difficulties and lasting damage.

Signs Your Vagal Nerve Is Powerless

Vagal nerve sign can wind up feeble or the nerve can move toward becoming bothered because of overwhelming metal poisonous quality, poor stance, Hiatal hernias, abundance liquor, stress, and mind injury (a solitary blackout can cause powerless vagal nerve tone). Indications of powerless vagal nerve tone or misregulated terminating of the vagal nerve can cause the accompanying manifestations:

- Lack of a muffle reflex

- Slow absorption nourishment sits in your stomach excessively long. This can cause heartburn or GERD, swelling, or clogging.

- Inability to unwind

- Heart palpitations

- Insomnia

Probably the best indication of solid vagal tone is the point at which your pulse increments somewhat with inward breath, and moderate marginally with exhalation.

How would you reinforce the vagal nerve?

About 60% of vagal nerve tone is dictated by hereditary qualities, however there is a strong 40% that we can affect! Become familiar with various approaches to fortify and animate the vagus nerve.

Fun truth: you CAN overstimulate the vagus nerve, and this is the most widely recognized reason for blacking out. If you've at any point blacked out or felt tipsy in the wake of giving blood or getting a shot, you likely experienced "vasovagal syncope". At the point when you are under exceptionally high pressure your vagus nerve turns out to be excessively invigorated and your pulse drops rapidly making you feel woozy or lose cognizance. It's just brief, and sitting or resting for the most part settle the inclination rapidly. No harm has been done don't as well, stress!

Frail vagal nerve tone is connected to aggravation, wretchedness, forlornness and cardiovascular failures. We need to ensure our vagal nerves are solid! The accompanying all invigorate the vagus nerve only enough to be exceptionally restorative, however less to cause blacking out but rather more these are not profoundly distressing occasions.

1. Gargling

Gargling animates the vagus nerve, albeit dainty swishing won't do it. You have to wash noisily and forcefully, to the point of nearly choking. Doing this day by day will help increment the responsiveness of your vagal nerve to direct unwinding, absorption, digestion and that's just the beginning.

2.Playing instruments

Fascinating research with didgeridoos demonstrated that playing the instrument is compelling in treating obstructive rest issue and rest apnea through its solid incitement of the vagus nerve. Further research demonstrates that various provocative conditions additionally improved. Most wind instruments animate the vagus nerve.

3.Yogic or Deep Breathing

Holding your breath for 6-8 checks animates the vagus nerve. Attempt this: Use your stomach to take in for a check of 6, hold for 6-8, and breathe out gradually through pressed together lips for 6-8 tallies to get your vagus terminating. It's essential to have the option to feel your stomach (that line between your stomach and ribs) going all over with every breath. It takes around 10 minutes of this breathing to feel the profoundly loosening up impacts of the vagal nerve incitement.

4.Meditation

Learning cherishing graciousness reflections improves vagal tone. This is because of its impact on positive feelings and positive associations. There increasingly positive feelings and associations we have, the more grounded our vagal tone. Download my free reflection present.

5. Acupuncture

Acupuncture is astonishing for managing vagal nerve reaction. At my office, I've built up an exceptionally powerful strategy utilizing electroacupuncture on explicit ear and body focuses that animate the vagus nerve to fortify tone and control vagal reaction. Electroacupuncture utilizes a little machine that emanates an effortless electromagnetic heartbeat. The electromagnetic heartbeat feels like a slight humming or tapping and isn't horrendous. Following 20-30 minutes of this, you will leave the workplace feeling unbelievably loose. That vagal nerve incitement will help direct every one of the procedures constrained by the vagal nerve, which at this point you know is a whoop dee doo! Would you be able to detect the needle therapy focuses in the photograph above?

Bioelectronics is a developing field of medication where little gadgets are embedded to animate diverse sensory system pathways. This effectively treats a scope of maladies and provocative side effects. This is energizing and approving of needle therapy which uses needles and here and there power to invigorate the sensory system at various focuses to treat a scope of illness and incendiary side effects. If you need to be on the bleeding edge of logical research, and stay away from medical procedure to embed a metal gadget attempt the less intrusive way, needle therapy.

Chapter 6 Vagal Tone

There has been a lot of research into the vagus nerve and its connection to a person's mental as well as physical health. Research shows that a vagus nerve that exhibits a high vagal tone has a positive impact on a person's mood as well as their physical well-being.

A well-toned vagus nerve will quickly return the body back to its normal or relaxed state after it has had a stressful encounter. This happens because the vagal nerve quickly reduces the heart rate, blood pressure, stress levels, has a positive impact on the brain and encourages healthy digestion when it slows to its relaxed state.

Research has even found that if a pregnant mother has a low vagal tone when her child is born, the child too will have a low vagal tone. The infant may also have lower levels of serotonin and dopamine than normal.

The Vagal Tone Index Of The Vagus Nerve

Just like anything in the body the vagus nerve can get damaged, it can also overreact, and it can send faulty signals to the brain, i.e., it becomes dysfunctional.

The vagus nerve not only takes messages from the brain to the internal organs but also delivers messages from the internal organs to the brain. This means not only does the brain have control over the vagus nerve, but the nerve, in turn, can have an effect on brain function.

For example, there may be a bacterial infection in an organ regulated by the vagus nerve. The nerves in the organ send a message which is carried by the vagus nerve to the brain which causes it to affect a person's mood — you may feel horrible, sleepy, and just plain miserable.

As it is a long nerve that touches many parts of the body, there are many places that something can go wrong and cause a dysfunction of the vagus nerve. These places can be categorized according to the three main functions of the vagus nerve that can be susceptible to dysfunction.

Three Main Functions of the Vagus Nerve Susceptible to Dysfunction

- Direct communication to the brain.

- Delivering information from the brain to organs in the body.

- Delivering information for the organs in the body to the brain.

Signs and Symptoms of Vagus Nerve Dysfunction

- Aggressive behavior

There is nothing wrong with a bit of healthy aggression now and then. Especially when a person is being attacked. The problem is when there is a constant display of aggression.

Usually, when aggressive behavior is triggered the body is able to calm itself down. If there is a dysfunction in the vagal nerve however, the body constantly thinks it is under threat and so it keeps the body in its fight or flight mode.

- Anxiety

Everyone experiences a bit of anxiety, in this fast-paced world it is hard not to have some form of stress or pressure pushing down on you. A healthy vagus nerve has the ability to counteract the fight or flight mode caused by stress and calm the body back down to a normal state.

If a person is in a constant state of anxiety, the sympathetic nervous system keeps triggering hormones to help the body defend itself. However, the body can only tolerate a certain amount of these hormones before it starts to be severely affected by them. Just like you would be if you took too much of any substance.

- Depression

Depression is a hard disorder to control and manage as it causes a person to be in a constant state of feeling down, blue, sad, and to lose interest in just about everything. It can cause a person to behave erratically, have bad mood swings, and even contemplate or attempt suicide.

There are various processes in the brain that influence depressive disorders, and the vagus nerve is one of the influencers. But just as it can influence depression, studies have shown it can also help to alleviate depression.

- Emotional

When the vagus nerve is not working properly it affects your emotions. One minute you will feel fine, but the next you will feel all teary or you may get angry. If the body is stuck in the fight or flight mode it will keep releasing hormones, eventually, it is going to take a toll on your system. It can present as a person being over-emotional.

- Painful inflamed joints

The vagus nerve is part of the system that prevents inflammation by alerting the brain to the substances that cause inflammation. This then lets the brain send signals to the system that is responsible for fighting off the inflammation. If the vagus nerve is not functioning correctly, it cannot get this signal to the brain to fight proinflammatory cytokines so it cannot stop the inflammation reflex.

- Constantly feeling dizzy

If the vagus nerve is overstimulated it can drop the blood pressure or heart rate too low which can cause a person to feel dizzy and even in some cases faint. The vagus nerve is responsible for the constriction of blood vessels in order to slow down the heart rate and lower blood pressure after a stressful situation for the body.

- Tired all the time

When any part of your body is not functioning well it takes a toll on your system. A person feeling tired when their body is sick or when something has gone wrong is the body's defense mechanism to help fight off illness or to try and right itself. As it does this best when a person is asleep, you will feel tired and miserable.

- Erratic heartbeat

As the vagus nerve controls the heart rate, one that is not working correctly could make your heartbeat increase and then drop suddenly. This makes motions like walking, standing, and even sitting up difficult to do.

- Irritable bowel syndrome, GERD, and indigestion

The vagus nerve is the nerve that sends a signal to tell the brain that the gut needs to get ready to digest food when a person starts to chew. The food we are chewing starts to get broken down and as we swallow various acids break it down even more so that it is easy to digest. A faulty vagus nerve can cause this movement to slow down so that food takes longer to digest. This means acid build-up, waste products, and partially digested food start to cause all sorts of complications for the system. These complications can manifest as irritable bowel syndrome, gastroesophageal reflux disease (GERD), heartburn, and acid indigestion.

- Passing out for no reason

When the vagus nerve is overstimulated, it constricts the blood vessels, cutting off blood flow to the brain. This causes a drop in heart rate and blood pressure which causes a person to pass out.

A dysfunctional vagus nerve may lead to a more serious condition if it is not treated. If you are exhibiting any of the signs above, you should seek advice from your doctor as if left untreated the issues can and probably will escalate.

Conditions That Could Arise from a Dysfunctional Vagus Nerve

- Dissociation
- Eating disorders
- Obsessive-compulsive disorder (OCD)
- Tinnitus
- Circulation problems
- Cluster and chronic migraine headaches
- Cancer
- Heart disease and chronic heart failure
- Leaky Gut Syndrome (LGS)
- Obesity
- Chronic mood swings
- Fibromyalgia

- A disorder that affects the memory such as Alzheimer's

The dysfunction of the vagal nerve or even damage to it is usually associated with lifestyle choices, disease, or physical damage to the nerve itself.

Diseases and Lifestyle Choices That Can Cause Dysfunction or Damage the Vagus Nerve

- Diabetes

Diabetes causes fluctuations in blood glucose levels which can damage the vagus nerve. This can lead to gastric problems as the vagus nerve controls how quickly the stomach gets emptied and diabetic damage to the nerve can cause gastroparesis. Gastroparesis is when the stomach does not empty completely.

- Chronic fatigue syndrome and Fibromyalgia

If the vagus nerve is dysfunctional or becomes damaged, it may misinterpret signals which can cause it to keep sending signals to the brain to shut down by sending out hormones that cause fatigue and pain.

- Poor posture

This can lead to constriction of the vagus nerve, which in turn, can lead to all sorts of physical problems such as poor digestion. This can lead to other internal problems for the system. Poor posture also leads to poor breathing and not getting enough oxygen into the blood can affect the vagus tone index.

- Chronic stress and anxiety

Chronic stress constantly puts pressure on the parasympathetic and sympathetic systems. The system will be in a constant state of switching on mobilization mode and then trying to switch off mobilization mode to bring the body back to normal. A state of constant stress is like flicking a light bulb on and off all the time, eventually, the bulb is going to blow. This is the same for people who are anxious all the time and live with constant worries that they cannot shut off.

- Smoking

Smoking causes a lot of problems for the nervous system. It damages the vagus nerve and the way it responds to cardiac signals, it also affects the lungs and other organs that the vagus nerve is responsible for.

- Excessive intake of alcohol

When the body consumes alcohol, it inhibits certain receptors in the brain, which causes vagal neuropathy. It reduces cardiac vagal tone which if continued to be abused will start to have serious effects on the rest of the nerve. As the nerve touches many organs in the body it could have a knock-on effect.

- Physical damage to any part of the vagus nerve

If parts of the vagus nerve get damaged it can cause serious mental and physical issues. The nerve can be damaged through injury or by various diseases. Seizures have been known to cause damage to the vagus nerve

In order to help the nerve recover or keep it healthy, a person needs to consider their lifestyle and commit to making some changes in order to improve their quality of life by increasing their vagal tone index. Vagal tone represents the activity of the vagus nerve, the better the tone, the faster the body reverts back to a normal or relaxed state from a stressful situation.

Chapter 7 Health And Life Benefits

The vagus nerve, when used to its full potential, can have extremely positive effects in combating a host of physical and mental diseases, including migraines, depression, PTSD, inflammation, trauma, fibromyalgia, and a number of other diseases. Yes, mental illness is very much real and has physical components that come from it. It is not simply a thinking disease. We will break down the various diseases individually and discuss how the vagus nerve can be used to positively affect them.

We have really gotten in-depth on what the vagus nerve is, what it does, how it relates to the rest of the body, and how stimulating it can have immense health benefits and improve our overall well-being. We also described in detail what the effects of an unhealthy vagus nerve are. For this reason, we must do our best to keep the vagus nerve healthy. The vagus nerve is a critical juncture in the human body, and it cannot be ignored when trying to improve health and avoid disease. Continued research on the vagus nerve has shown that utilizing it to its full ability will be a great benefit to anyone who is willing to harness it. While you may not have known much about the vagus nerve before starting this book, we hope that you know more about it now. Since we understand how many physiological processes the nerve moderates. We will now get into how many illnesses it can improve.

Vagus Nerve And Migraines

Migraines, for lack of a better phrase, really create a headache for us. They can really slow us down and impact our lifestyles. Many people suffer from migraines to the point they need to seek medical help and even get admitted to the hospital. Think about how a headache makes you feel. A bad enough headache will make you feel like you don't want to do anything at all. They negatively affect your activities of daily living, and having one every day would be like torture. Migraines are basically a recurring headache. They often occur on one side of the head, create a throbbing sensation, and may have a genetic predisposition. This is true for a small percentage of the population. Migraines can also be triggered by things like smells, lights, noises, certain foods, medication, lack of sleep, alcohol, tobacco use and a wealth of other sources. Whatever the cause of a migraine may be, they are absolutely no fun to have, and if we can help eliminate them in some way, it will absolutely benefit many people. No matter how big and tough you are, a bad migraine can put you out of commission easily. It is a pain even the toughest among us cannot handle for too long.

The vagus nerve can be used to help eliminate or reduce migraines significantly. The best part is, we all have a vagus nerve and can use it. The case is still out on whether vagus nerve stimulation can help with migraines. However, several research studies show that people who received vagus nerve stimulation over multiple years reported a significant improvement in their migraines. This was both in frequency and pain level. A survey that was conducted by Southern Illinois University for individuals who received vagus nerve stimulation for epilepsy, also showed that multiple people who had migraines prior to the therapy reported vast improvements in frequency and pain levels. Basically, all of the people who did have migraines prior to the therapies report vast improvements afterward. This is a strong indication that vagus nerve stimulation significantly impacts migraines in a positive way. Of course, these stimulations were done medically using implanted devices. However, many of the techniques we can still have minor, indirect effects.

Many other prominent studies have shown that stimulation of the vagus nerve, including the noninvasive approach, significantly reduced migraines for a large number of individuals. This further cements that direct nerve stimulation is not necessary to help reduce migraines. The reporting in the reduction of pain is done by the patients themselves, which is really the strongest indication. If a person states they are not in pain, then they are not in pain. Many of these individuals also reported a higher quality of life due to the lack of pain. When a person has less pain, they are more likely to continue healthy practices as well.

A study done by a prominent neurologist in the early 2000s discusses a patient he had with chronic epileptic seizures. Unfortunately, for whatever reason, the Vagus nerve stimulation did not improve epilepsy. Not every therapy will work for every individual as each human organism is unique in its own way. This was an unfortunate circumstance for this patient. However, they were surprised to learn that the patient had a major reduction in his chronic migraines. Much to the joy of the patient. This was not the intended result, but since it worked, the treatment was partially successful. Researchers are continuing to do further studies on this phenomenon between the vagus nerve and migraines. It was really found by accident as multiple people who were getting treated for seizures using stimulation, surprisingly had an improvement in their migraines and headaches. The parasympathetic response of the vagus nerve seems to significantly reduce and even eliminate the causes of severe migraines. The parasympathetic response likely inhibits the overstimulation of the sympathetic nervous system in these cases, effectively altering the pain response. Vagus nerve stimulation also reduces stress, which can be a trigger for migraines. When the sympathetic nervous system is elevated, stress is increased. When the parasympathetic inhibitory response kicks in, stress, and in turn, pain, is significantly decreased

Next time that migraine hits try some of the techniques we earlier. Go for a long walk or hit the gym. This may be difficult as exercise will be the last thing on your mind. As well, you can simply sit and take some deep breaths, hum or take a cold shower. Whatever you can do, try it out. Stimulating and utilizing the full potential of the vagus nerve can vastly improve migraines and improve your quality of life.

Vagus Nerve And Depression

Depression, or major depressive disorder, is a mood disorder that causes a person to have persistent feelings of sadness and loss of interest. Depression can affect a person both mentally and physically and take a major toll on a person's daily activities. It is an illness, just like any other, that can cause a person to just not want to face life and become secluded. Even though mental health is gaining prominence and becoming accepted by the general population, there is still a major segment of the population that does not take it seriously. They feel that a person can just snap out of it. This is not the case. A person cannot just snap out of it. Depression is more than just getting over something. It is an illness that may require medical attention. There is a difference between having an off day, and a major depressive disorder that significantly reduces your ability to function every single day. When a person is suffering from severe depression, they are often walking a thin line, and one little thing could push them over the edge. For this reason, their feelings and mood disorders always need to be validated. They need to be taken seriously.

Untreated depression can lead to extensive pain and trauma. Severe depression may lead to a person harming themselves. There are many unfortunate stories of people who did not reach out for help, out of fear of appearing weak, and things took a turn for the worse. We do not want this to happen to anybody because they felt like they could not reach out to someone. Depression is not something to take lightly, and if a person is exhibiting the signs of depression, it must be taken very seriously. There are many signs and symptoms of depression that must be considered. Among them are feelings of sadness and tearfulness, anxiety, reduced appetite, unexplained physical problems, feelings of worthlessness, seclusion, loss of interest, anger, frustration, always blaming themselves, and many other things. Take special notice when someone suddenly stops doing something they have always loved to do. Also, give special attention to major mood swings.

A study conducted in 2002 in biological psychiatry showcased outcomes that long term vagus nerve stimulation vastly improved symptoms of major depressive disorder and reduced episodes of depression. Stimulation of the vagus nerve appears to change brain wave patterns, which reduces the symptoms of depression. This implies a significant physical component for depression. However, doctors are still not fully aware of exactly how vagus nerve stimulation improves symptoms of depression. It just seems to work well, which is a good thing. Perhaps there is a connection between an overstimulated sympathetic nervous system, which speeds up body processes and depression. This is something that is still not fully understood. One thing that researchers want to emphasize is that stimulating the vagus nerve may not eliminate depression completely, but it will still vastly improve a person's quality of life. If a person can at least feel good the majority of the time, then a particular therapy is worth giving attention to.

Next time a person you know and love is experiencing symptoms of depression, don't get annoyed. Depression is an illness, just like diabetes, and a person suffering from it needs support, and not be told to just get over it. Perhaps using the natural techniques for vagus nerve stimulation may be beneficial for them. Once again, it may not cure their depression, but it will improve their mood and ability to live life tremendously. If vagus nerve stimulation continues to effectively inhibit depression, then maybe the stigma that still exists around mental illness can be eliminated once and for all. This just may be the greatest result of all. Even people who suffer from mental illness feel guilty. We don't hear people apologizing for heart disease. But they still apologize for being depressed. This needs to stop, and increased vagus nerve research can help.

Here is one suggestion that will help all parties involved. When helping a friend who is experiencing depression, take them out to have some fun. Remember that laughing and having a good time helps to stimulate the vagus nerve. Take your friend out for a night on the town, and you may just help with their depression.

Vagus Nerve And PTSD

Post-Traumatic Stress Disorder, or PTSD, is a mental condition caused by a traumatic event that had a severe impact on someone. The people who are affected most commonly are in the military, law enforcement, first responders, or anyone in a field where tragedy is a common occurrence. However, PTSD may also strike just about anybody and everybody who has been through a traumatic event. A serious accident, death of a loved one, getting assaulted or any number of tragic events may cause a person to have PTSD. It may take years to overcome PTSD and some never overcome it at all. PTSD can manifest itself in multiple ways, including anxiety, anger, nervousness, negative thoughts, flashbacks, and chronic pain. They will often reexperience the trauma multiple times in their heads. There is a major split, even within the military community, whether or not PTSD is legitimate or not. For this reason, just like with depression, people will dismiss it as a non-issue. They believe that someone can just get over it. A person cannot just get over it though. PTSD is very real and is a serious mental disorder that needs to be treated as such. Unfortunately, PTSD continues to carry a negative stigma to it that can hopefully be a thing of the past once people start realizing some of the physical elements to it as well.

While there is no known cure for PTSD, there are therapies that may be used to help subside some of the signs and symptoms. Currently, some of the therapies include talk therapy and exposure therapy. Several studies suggest that vagus nerve stimulation may be a productive adjunct therapy for helping with PTSD, especially with the pain that is associated with it. A University of Texas, Dallas, study researched the effects of vagus nerve stimulation on rats. The rats in this particular study were shown to display some signs that come with PTSD, like fear, aggression, and anxiety. A session of vagus nerve stimulation showed a significant reduction in these negative signs. Not only that, the signs did not return in many cases after another episode of trauma, suggesting that the stimulation may have more long-term effects than the other therapies. Researchers feel that if the stimulation can work in the same manner in humans, it may significantly reduce the pain associated with PTSD. If the effects are more long term as well, then it is certainly an adjunct therapy worth looking into.

If you have a friend or loved one who experiences PTSD, perhaps it is time to get to work on them. Help them by using the techniques that will stimulate their vagus nerve. That old cliché of "laughter is the best medicine" may be the ultimate tool in this situation. Help your loved one get regular exercise. Remember, this does not just mean going to the gym. Most people are more likely to do something if they enjoy it. Find something they want to do physically and help them do it. If they love playing basketball, play a quick pickup game. If they love going for walks, find a nice trail, and enjoy the sites. Whatever you can do to get them moving, do it. Finally, how about a nice round of karaoke? Singing and dancing are definitely a great way to stimulate the vagus nerve and get your friends out of the poor mental state they are in. If we can continue to correlate vagus nerve stimulation with helping to subside the signs of PTSD, then hopefully, we can remove the stigma associated with it as well. Just like with depression, we may never be able to cure PTSD, but we can certainly manage it with the appropriate practices.

We want to talk further about how PTSD can manifest itself into physical symptoms like muscle tightness, chest pain, fatigue, and digestive issues. Many of these physical responses to a traumatic event indicate a sympathetic nervous system activity. Things like muscle tightness and chest pain that is not heart-related often come from stress and being worked up for so long. They do not come from being in a relaxed state. Furthermore, fatigue develops when the body is overly stressed for long periods of time. This is why excessive sympathetic responses are not healthy for the body. If your body is in a constant state of pain and tiredness due to a traumatic event, then perhaps it is time to really start stimulating your vagus nerve to inactivate your parasympathetic response. The inhibition from the parasympathetic response will put your body in a state of relaxation, releasing the built-up tension and helping to reduce the pain associated with PTSD. Do this regularly, and it can really help to manage the negative signs and symptoms of Post-Traumatic Stress Disorder.

Vagus Nerve And Inflammation

Does the vagus nerve help with inflammation? Yes, it does. Inflammation, also known as the inflammatory response, is your body's natural response to a variety of things, such as stress. The inflammatory response occurs under many circumstances, especially when our body is trying to fight off disease. Mild inflammation is needed for the body to maintain its proper functions. When the body perceives some type of threat, like an illness or injury, the inflammatory response kicks in to subdue the threat. This can be marked by swelling, pain, fevers, and fatigue. Once again, inflammation is needed to help out bodies maintain their functionality. However, excessive or untreated inflammation can create many health problems throughout the body. In cases of stress, inflammation may occur due to the fight or flight response of the sympathetic nervous system. In general, whenever the body perceives any type of threat, it inhibits the parasympathetic nervous system and stimulates the sympathetic response so that it can deal with the perceived threat. This is why you will notice an increase in heart rate when a person has an infection.

The body is becoming stimulated in order to defend itself.

Since the vagus nerve is the main component of the parasympathetic nervous system, proper stimulation will help to counteract the sympathetic nervous system, effectively reducing inflammation. Especially in the case of inflammation, which can occur for a number of reasons, stimulating the vagus nerve on a regular basis is of great importance. While there are many other interventions that may need to be done to combat chronic inflammation, exercises to stimulate and activate the vagus nerve are an appropriate adjunct therapy to help suppress the sympathetic nervous. An excessive, heightened response will eventually have detrimental health consequences. The vagus nerve's ability to control inflammation through the parasympathetic response showcases its ability to indirectly affect the immune system, which produces the inflammatory response mechanism.

Stress is a major trigger for the inflammatory response also. Indicating even further, the sympathetic nervous system is at play here. In this case, things like deep breathing and humming will effectively reduce stress, inhibit the sympathetic response, stimulate the vagus nerve and ultimately reduce inflammation. The vagus nerve, when stimulated to its full potential, can strongly influence the immune system, thereby influencing good health. The vagus nerve is looking stronger and stronger the more we talk about it.

Vagus Nerve and Fibromyalgia

Fibromyalgia is a disorder characterized by widespread musculoskeletal pain. It is often accompanied by fatigue, sleep issues, and mood dysfunction. There is still not much known about fibromyalgia as the pain does not come from a specific cause or area in the body. Many researchers believe that with fibromyalgia, painful sensations are amplified due to the way the brain processes pain. A true cause is not fully known at this juncture.

Sometimes the pain is triggered by a certain event, like an accident or surgery. Other times, there is no single event, but the pain just seems to accumulate over time. There is no cure for fibromyalgia at this moment. However, there are interventions, both medical and nonmedical, that can help with subsiding the symptoms that come with it. Once again, our friend, the vagus nerve, is at play here.

In a 2011 NIH study, they suggested that vagus nerve stimulation may be a useful adjunct treatment for patients with fibromyalgia. Further research was definitely needed, though. Many researchers feel that vagus nerve stimulation is effective in treating pain because it is able to negate a wide variety of factors that contribute to pain, like inflammation and the pain response. There is still much that is up in the air about fibromyalgia. However, the results of studies continue to suggest that the pain associated with it is significantly reduced with vagus nerve stimulation. Pain is often heightened during times when the body is at stress. Since the vagus nerve can lower a person's stress through the sympathetic response, it is reasonable to believe it can reduce or even eliminate pain associated with fibromyalgia.

Vagus Nerve And Epilepsy

We have been mentioning epilepsy, or seizure disorder, throughout this portion of the book. Namely, because it was the main disorder that was targeted by vagus nerve stimulation for being able to be cured with the proper techniques. Furthermore, many positive benefits of vagus nerve stimulation were discovered, while researchers were studying the effects of it with epilepsy. Epilepsy is a major central nervous disorder in which brain activity becomes exceedingly abnormal, causing seizures or periods of very unusual behavior. The nerves and neurons are firing uncontrollably, causing erratic and uncontrollable movements. A person who suffers from epilepsy has their whole world turned upside down due to the severity of the condition and the way it takes over their life. A person will often never know when a seizure will hit, and this can prevent them from doing many activities like driving. It will also inhibit their ability to go into certain professions. It is a very dangerous and stressful disease to have to deal with.

During an epileptic episode, the sympathetic nervous system is in complete overdrive, causing excessive and erratic movements within the nervous system. When a person is having a full-blown epileptic attack or seizure, we probably won't be able to attempt the many stimulating practices we went over. Much more extreme measures will need to be taken. However, what can be done is the vagal tone can be strengthened to help avoid or reduce epileptic attacks in the future. The stronger the vagal tone, the better adept the parasympathetic response will be, and the better it will become at inhibiting the sympathetic response. We mentioned before how massaging the carotid sinus has been shown to inhibit seizure activity by stimulating the vagus nerve. If this technique can work, then it is a good indication that the other techniques will also.

The goal overall is to continuously improve and strengthen the vagus nerve as much as possible. We will not be able to prevent or cure all illnesses. However, as we strengthen our own vagal tone, we can help to improve the functionality of the body and at least prevent or reduce many diseases. The point of vagus nerve stimulation is to keep it healthy, active, and strong so that it has the ability to enhance parasympathetic activity as much as possible. When we increase our body's ability to utilize the parasympathetic response, we will be able to effectively reduce seizure activity.

Most of the research behind vagus nerve stimulation has been to help prevent epilepsy. This suggests that it is still considered a strong therapy in inhibiting seizure activity.

The Vagus Nerve "Helps"

One of the words we have used constantly throughout this book is the word "help." We have said that the vagus nerve "helps" the human body. We say this because the vagus nerve alone cannot just solve all of our problems.

At least, not at this moment. Stimulating and utilizing the power of the vagus nerve is more of an adjunct therapy for helping to improve body processes and prevent chronic diseases, both physical and mental. We don't want it to sound like a cure-all. Of course, it will cure a lot. Allow your vagus nerve to "help" you feel better. The point is to make the vagus nerve work as efficiently for us as possible.

Chapter 8 Vagus Nerve: Its Importance To Weight Loss And Health

Have you at any point asked why a few people feel full in the wake of eating a limited quantity of nourishment and other individuals are as yet hungry until they eat a major serving?

The appropriate response may be in the affectability of their vagus nerve. The vagus nerve is the nerve that associates your gut to your mind, and it's a significant piece of the parasympathetic sensory system (the "rest and summary" reaction, essentially something contrary to "battle or flight").

•All signals going up from the gut to the mind through the vagus nerve influences your possibility of totality or more cravings, your disposition and feelings of anxiety, and the initiation of your provocative pressure reaction.

•Signals running down the vagus nerve from the cerebrum to the gut influence assimilation, discharge of stomach related compounds, and gastrointestinal motility (that is an extravagant word for where you are on the scale from clogging to looseness of the bowels).

It's an extremely significant pathway, and vagus nerve initiation is associated with stoutness, gastrointestinal illnesses, cardiovascular sicknesses, disposition issue like despondency, and a wide range of other incessant medical issues. Here's a glance at why the vagus nerve is so significant, and how your eating routine can improve your wellbeing by influencing vagal nerve signals from the gut.

The Vagus Nerve And Hunger

One extremely significant kind of correspondence that keeps running here and there the vagus nerve is craving and totality signals. For instance...

•The physical greater part of nourishment in the stomach sends satiety flag up the vagus nerve to your mind. This is the manner by which your mind knows to quit feeling hungry after a supper.

•Nutrient detecting and synapses delivered in the gut, similar to serotonin and ghrelin, can likewise send yearning and totality flag up the vagus nerve to the cerebrum.

Corpulence is related with a lower affectability of the vagus nerve to completion signals, and there's a great deal of proof this is caused explicitly by eating routine.

Heftiness inciting diets can really adjust the affectability of the vagus nerve to completion signals, so it takes more nourishment for your cerebrum to get the "full presently" signal. Also, much the same as you may expect, invigorating the vagus nerve (to "increase the volume" on the satiety signal) will in general reason weight reduction in test creatures – despite the fact that it's significant that reviews in people have blended outcomes.

The Vagus Nerve and Other Health Issues

Appetite is one integral motivation behind why the vagus nerve is significant. However, in the event that you bring a jump into PubMed, you'll see that vagus nerve brokenness is really connected with a wide range of different issues. That is on the grounds that the vagus nerve likewise manages irritation, and aggravation is engaged with pretty much every ceaseless malady. Invigorating vagus nerve sign to the cerebrum is calming – it flag the mind to turn down the pressure reaction and lessen the generation of incendiary cytokines.

The impacts here are somewhat difficult to unravel in light of the fact that the vagus nerve is a two-way road and there are a ton of convoluted input circles between the cerebrum and the gut (recall that the vagus nerve runs the two different ways!). Be that as it may, for individuals who simply care about improving their wellbeing, the accurate system may be less significant than the outcomes, which are certainly noteworthy:

•Vagus nerve control of irritation influences cardiovascular wellbeing, and vagus nerve incitement may help counteract cardiovascular occasions.

•Vagus nerve flagging is lost in patients with Crohn's Disease (a type of Inflammatory Bowel Disease), and one little, starter concentrate found that vagal nerve incitement helps treat the indications.

•The vagus nerve may likewise be engaged with Irritable Bowel Syndrome, and vagal incitement may be useful for diminishing IBS torment.

•This study is truly intriguing: treating diabetes-inclined rodents with vagal nerve incitement forestalls both sorrow and insulin obstruction. That is a gigantic bit of proof that downturn and diabetes may both have establishes in the gut.

On the off chance that a terrible eating routine is influencing the affectability of your vagus nerve, it could likewise significantly affect every one of these ailments.

This could be one motivation behind why gut wellbeing is such a major player in generally speaking wellbeing.

Care and Feeding of your Vagus Nerve

Up until now, we realize that an obesogenic "cafeteria diet" (high-fat, high-carb shoddy nourishment) diminishes the affectability of the vagus nerve, and that vagus nerve incitement neutralizes that, with enormous advantages for weight... and for pretty much everything else. Lamentably, the "vagal nerve incitement" in these examinations isn't something you can do at home; it's a gadget that the subjects got carefully embedded in their bodies.

However, on the off chance that a lousy eating routine can lessen the affectability of the vagus nerve, possibly a decent diet can help reestablish it. Other than "don't eat a low quality nourishment diet," here's somewhat progressively explicit research.

This examination found that dietary fat decreased aggravation through its impacts on the vagus nerve. The creators inferred that "high-fat... sustenance is possibly remedial in different fiery issue, for example, sepsis and provocative gut infection (IBD) portrayed by an incendiary reaction in which... intestinal obstruction capacity is disabled."

That is upheld up by the association between a ketogenic (exceptionally high-fat, low-carb) diet and vagal nerve incitement as two viable treatments for treatment-safe epilepsy. It's conceivable that a ketogenic diet have a portion of its craving stifling, calming impacts through invigorating the vagus nerve.

This investigation additionally found that a probiotic (Lactobacillus casei strain Shirota) actuated the vagus nerve. The probiotic changed the gut-to-cerebrum stress motioning in understudies taking a distressing test and stifled the arrival of the pressure hormone cortisol. That proposes that probiotics may have the option to break the gut-cerebrum gut-mind input cycle here and there the vagus nerve where mental pressure messes gut up, which send increasingly hormonal pressure sign to the cerebrum, which cause more gut issues.

High-impact exercise may likewise be useful.

For moment satisfaction, you can likewise do your very own vagal nerve incitement utilizing the Valsalva move. Plunk down, in light of the fact that it can make you somewhat dazed. Take a full breath, and afterward close your mouth and squeeze your nose shut with the goal that no air can get away. At that point imagine like you're attempting to inhale out, yet without opening your nose or mouth – you should feel the weight from the air. Continue doing this for 15-20 seconds, and afterward let the let some circulation into and inhale typically. (On the off chance that you do any weightlifting, this is the kind of breath-holding you do to settle your spine during overwhelming squats and deadlifts.)

The Valsalva move doesn't have long haul impacts, however it may be useful for a prompt circumstance, similar to directly before a test or in an unpleasant drive.

That is not a great deal to go on – there simply aren't numerous investigations on eating regimen and the vagus nerve. In any case, it's something to begin with, and it backs up the significant ways that the gut, the mind, and the remainder of your body are altogether associated. Thinking about the vagus nerve clarifies why gut wellbeing, psychological wellness, and entire body wellbeing are so tangled up with one another, and why great gut wellbeing is so significant for things route past processing.

Chapter 9 Vagus Nerve Stimulation Techniques

The vagus nerve shouldn't be stunned into shape. It can likewise be conditioned and fortified like a muscle. Here are some straightforward things you can do that may improve your wellbeing notably:

1. Positive Social Relationships – An investigation had members ponder others while quietly rehashing positive expressions about loved ones. Contrasted with the controls, the meditators demonstrated a general increment in positive feelings like quietness, euphoria, and expectation in the wake of finishing the class. These positive musings of others prompted an improvement in the vagal capacity, as found in pulse fluctuation. The outcomes additionally demonstrated a more conditioned vagus nerve than when just thinking.

2. Cold – "Cold presentation, for example, chilly showers or face dunking invigorates the nerve also," says Mentor.

Studies demonstrate that when your body acclimates to chilly, your battle or flight (thoughtful) framework decreases, and your rest and review (parasympathetic) framework increments, and this is interceded by the vagus nerve. Any excellent cold presentation, including drinking super cold water, will expand vagus nerve actuation.

    3. Rinsing – Another home solution for an under-invigorated vagus nerve is to swish with water. Rinsing invigorates the muscles of the bed, which are terminated by the vagus nerve.

"Commonly, patients will tear up a piece which is a decent sign, and if they don't, we suggest that they do it consistently until they see that they do fire destroying a piece," says Hoffman. "This has been appeared to promptly improve working memory execution."

    4. Singing And Chanting – Humming, mantra reciting, psalm-singing, and playful, enthusiastic singing all expansion pulse inconstancy (HRV) in somewhat various ways. Song resembles starting a vagal siphon conveying loosening up waves. Singing as loud as possible works the muscles in the back of the throat to initiate the vagus. Singing as one,

which is regularly done in temples and synagogues, additionally expands HRV and vagus work. Singing has been found to expand oxytocin, otherwise called the adoration hormone, since it makes individuals feel more like each other.

5. Back rub – You can invigorate your vagus nerve by rubbing your feet and your neck along the carotid sinus, situated along the carotid supply routes on either side of your neck. A neck back rub can help lessen seizures. A foot back rub help can bring down your pulse and circulatory strain. A weight back rub can likewise actuate the vagus nerve. These back rubs are utilised to enable newborn children to put on weight by animating gut work, generally interceded by actuating the vagus nerve.

6. Giggling – Happiness and chuckling are characteristic invulnerable sponsors. Chuckling likewise invigorates the vagus nerve. Research demonstrates how chuckling builds HRV in a gathering domain.

There are different case reports of individuals blacking out from giggling, and this might be from the vagus nerve/parasympathetic framework being animated excessively. Swooning can come after laughing just as pee, hacking, gulping, or stable discharge—which are all aided along by vagus enactment.

7. Yoga And Tai Chi — Both increment vagus nerve movement and your parasympathetic framework all in all. Studies have demonstrated that yoga expands GABA, a quieting synapse in your mind. Analysts trust it does this by "invigorating vagal afferents (strands)," which increment action in the parasympathetic sensory system. This is particularly useful for individuals who battle with tension or misery.

8. Breathing Deeply And Slowly — Your heart and neck contain neurons that have receptors called baroreceptors, which identify pulse and transmit the neuronal sign to your cerebrum. This enacts your vagus nerve that associates with your heart to lower circulatory strain and vibration. Slow breathing, with a generic equivalent measure of time taking in and out,

builds the affectability of baroreceptors and vagal enactment. Breathing around 5-6 breaths for every moment in the average grown-up can be useful.

9. Exercise – Exercise expands your mind's development hormone, underpins your cerebrum's mitochondria, and helps turn around subjective decay. But at the same time, it's been showed to invigorate the vagus nerve, which prompts useful cerebrum and psychological wellness impacts. Gentle exercise likewise animates the gut stream, which is intervened by the vagus nerve.

10. Espresso Enemas — Enemas resemble dashes for your vagus nerve. Extending the entrail builds vagus nerve actuation, as is finished with purifications. This purging is cultivated by expanding the liver's ability to detoxify poisons in the blood and restricting them to the bile. All the while, the liver scrubs itself as it discharges the harmful bile into the little, at that point, an extensive, digestive system for clearing. The whole blood supply steam through the liver like clockwork. By holding the espresso 12 to 15 minutes, the blood will course four

to multiple times for purging, much like a dialysis treatment. The water substance of the espresso invigorates intestinal peristalsis and purges the digestive organ with the aggregated dangerous bile.

11. Nirvana — This wearable item sends a delicate electrical wave through the left ear waterway to animate the body's vagus nerve while matching up with music, which invigorates the arrival of synapses in the cerebrum that create a quieting sensation all through the body.

12. Unwind – Learning how to chill might be the No. 1 thing to help keep your vagus nerve conditioned. As indicated by Hoffman, most loosening up exercises will animate the vagus nerve.

Vagus Nerves Injure

It was imagined that vagal heartburn was brought about by vagal nerve brokenness brought about by damage to the vagus nerve damage related to intricacies of horrible reticuloperitonitis. It was guessed that the incendiary and scar tissue injuries influenced vagal nerve strands providing the forestomach and stomach. The ordinarily happening disorder was like the Hoflund disorder made by tentatively segmenting the vagus nerves, and therefore the expression "vagal acid reflux" was instituted.

The official clarification was that dorsal vagal nerve damage came about in achalasia of the reticuloomasal opening (front stenosis) and hindered the entry of ingesta from the reticulorumen into the omasum and stomach, bringing about a developed rumen with unusual rumen substance. Correspondingly, damage to the pyloric part of the ventral vagus nerve came about in achalasia of the pylorus (back stenosis) and hindered the progression of ingesta from the stomach bringing about abomasal impaction. The two irregularities brought about meagre defecation containing undigested long feed particles.

Be that as it may, even though as a rule of vagal heartburn, there are deep bonds between the reticulum and neighboring organs, there is little proof of vagal nerve damage. It is additionally realised that the disorder can happen with no gross evidence of irritation of the serosa of the forestomach and stomach over which the vagus nerves are found. Without gross sores, it has been proposed that tiny injuries of the average reticular divider where vagal strain receptors are found may meddle with forestomach motility and esophageal notch reflexes.

Different vagus nerve impacts include:

Correspondence between the cerebrum and the gut: The vagus nerve conveys data from the stomach to the mind.

Unwinding with profound breathing: The vagus nerve speaks with the stomach. With full breaths, an individual feel increasingly loose.

Diminishing irritation: The vagus nerve sends a mitigating sign to different pieces of the body.

Bringing down the pulse and circulatory strain: If the vagus nerve is overactive, it can prompt the heart being not able to siphon enough blood around the body. Sometimes, unreasonable vagus nerve action can cause loss of awareness and organ harm.

Dread administration: The vagus nerve sends data from the gut to the mind, which is connected to managing pressure, nervousness, and dread - consequently the maxim, "hunch." These sign assistance an individual to recoup from distressing and terrifying circumstances.

Vagus nerve Stimulation

Stimulation of the vagus nerve is a medicinal method that is utilised to attempt to treat an assortment of conditions. It tends to be done either physically or through electrical heartbeats.

The viability of vagus nerve incitement has been tried through clinical preliminaries. Thus, the United States Food and Drug Administration (FDA) has affirmed its utilisation to treat two distinct conditions.

Also, Vagal nerve stimulation is a treatment used to reduce the frequency and intensity of seizures when medications aren't effective.

The vagus nerve is one of many nerves that carry messages to and from the brain. It helps regulate internal organs such as the heart and stomach. Nerve fibres within the vagus nerve are connected to the part of the brain believed to be responsible for producing seizures.

This procedure involves placing a small electric stimulator in the neck around the vagus nerve and a power source near the armpit or chest. The device works like a heart pacemaker to stimulate the left vagus nerve. It automatically sends intermittent electrical signals to the brain and can be manually activated to attempt to interrupt a seizure that's just starting.

At UCSF Medical Center, our neurologists and neurosurgeons have expertise in implanting vagal nerve stimulators to treat seizures caused by diseases such as epilepsy.

Vagus nerve incitement includes the utilisation of a gadget to animate the vagus nerve with electrical driving forces. An implantable vagus nerve trigger is right now FDA-affirmed to treat epilepsy and sorrow. There's one vagus nerve on each area of your body, moving from your brainstem by your neck to your chest and stomach area.

In regular vagus nerve incitement, a gadget is precisely embedded under the skin on your chest, and a wire is strung under your skin, associating the device to one side vagus nerve. At the point when initiated, the tool sends an electrical flag along the left vagus nerve to your brainstem, which at that point, carries a sign to specific regions in your mind. The correct vagus nerve isn't utilised because it's bound to convey strands that supply nerves to the heart.

New, noninvasive vagus nerve incitement gadgets, which don't require careful implantation, have been endorsed in Europe to treat epilepsy, sadness, and agony. A noninvasive device that invigorates the vagus nerve was as of late approved by the Food and Drug Administration for the treatment of group cerebral pains in the United States.

Dependence on any substance can make the life of an individual upside down. From spending a fortune to deluding own family, an individual dependent on illicit substances can go to any degree. Be that as it may, how does habit power, somebody, to put such a significant amount in question and afterwards lose all? There are a few variables influencing everything with regards to managing the developing issue of fixation.

Longings are an extreme issue that torment various individuals battling illicit drug use, particularly when they attempt to fall off the addictive substance. Amusingly, numerous individuals would have effectively achieved long haul moderation if longings didn't manifest with habit. Aside from being considered as a significant impediment in recuperation treatment, desires are additionally the primary driver of backsliding.

Complete recuperation from dependence happens just when an individual is free from yearnings. Carrying on with a medication-free existence without the requirement for consistent observing against medication longings can be hard for a recuperating individual. However, an ongoing report distributed in the diary Learning and Memory has proposed that medication yearnings can be successfully treated with vagus nerve incitement (VNS) treatment. Under the procedure, the patients are shown new practices that supplant their old addictive conduct of looking for medications.

The job of VNS in enslavement recuperation in the University of Texas at Dallas study, the specialists, uncovered that the VNS treatment helped patients to recoup from the maladaptive conduct of medication taking. VNS is a careful procedure wherein a gadget is embedded to a wire strung along the vagus nerve, which goes up from the neck to the cerebrum and associates with the territory liable for controlling the state of mind. Estimated as little as a silver dollar, the gadget works simply like a pacemaker. It works by sending slight Electric heartbeats through the vagus nerve, which further reaches the mind, in this way controlling the desires and inclinations.

The approach is endorsed by the U.S. Nourishment and Drug Administration (FDA) and is considered as a potential treatment for treatment-safe sorrow, post-horrendous pressure issues (PTSD), and loss of motion. The investigation further featured that VNS encourages "annihilation learning" of medication looking for practices by diminishing desires and supplanting the activity related to dependence with new ones. "Eradication of dreadful recollections and termination of drugs looking for memories depends on a similar substrate in the cerebrum. In our trials, VNS encourages both the elimination learning and lessens the backslide reaction also.

Drug-free life is possible

Even though addictive substances prevail in incidentally easing enthusiastic and physical torments of medication abusers, they need to adapt to the disturbing manifestations of substance misuse in the long run. Other than building up a few physical and mental issues, a significant number of these people additionally become reckless and self-destructive.

Dependence on any substance can be hazardous. Just an extensive treatment program including detoxification, drugs, psychotherapies, and other experiential treatments like yoga, contemplation, and so on can enable a person to get calm. Also, a comprehensive recuperation of the executive's plan is similarly essential to support the time of balance and oversee longings. In any case, the degree to which human services specialists can accumulate brings about the treatment for illicit drug use is subject to the clinical qualities of the patients that may shift as indicated by the kind of medication being manhandled just as its amount, length and the technique for utilizing the prescription (oral or intravenous).

Five Vagus Nerve Stimulation Exercises

Except if you have a carefully embedded gadget, you really can't legitimately invigorate your vagus nerve; be that as it may, you can, by implication, animate your vagus nerve to assuage scratched up or shut down sensory system states. Keep in mind, and your vagus nerve goes through your stomach, stomach, lungs, throat, inward ear, and facial muscles. In this way, rehearses change or control the activities of these regions of the body can impact the working of the vagus nerve through the mind-body input circle. You can attempt these from the solace of your lounge room:

Murmuring:

The vagus nerve goes through by the vocal ropes, and the internal ear and the vibrations of murmuring is a free and straightforward approach to impact your sensory system states. Necessarily pick your preferred tune, and you're all set. Or then again, if yoga accommodates your way of life, you can "OM" your approach to prosperity. Notice and Appreciate the sensations in your chest, throat, and head.

Cognizant Breathing:

The breath is perhaps the quickest approach to impact our sensory system states. The point is to move the stomach and stomach with the inspiration and to hinder your relaxing. Vagus nerve incitement happens when the breathing is eased back from our run of the mill 10-14 breaths for every moment to 5-7 breaths for each moment. You can accomplish this by checking the inward breath to 5, hold quickly, and breathe out to a tally of 10. You can further invigorate the vagus nerve by making a slight choking at the back of the throat and making an "shh." Inhale like you are attempting to haze a mirror to make the inclination in the throat, however, breathe in and breathe out of the nose sound (in yoga, this is called Ujjayi Pranayam).

Valsalva Maneuver:

This convoluted name alludes to a procedure of endeavouring to breathe out against a shut aviation route. You can also do this by keeping your mouth shut and squeezing your nose while attempting to inhale out. This builds the weight within your chest pit, expanding vagal tone.

Jumping Reflex:

Considered a top-notch vagus nerve incitement method, sprinkling cold water all over from your lips to your scalp line invigorates the plunging reflex. You can likewise accomplish the sensory system cooling impacts by putting ice shapes in a ziplock and holding the ice against your face and a short hold of your breath. The jumping reflex eases back your pulse, builds bloodstream to your cerebrum, decreases outrage, and loosens up your body. A new procedure that invigorates the jumping reflex is to submerge your tongue in the fluid. Drink and hold heated water in your mouth, detecting the water with your language.

Association:

Reach out for relationships. Sound associations with others, regardless of whether this happens face to face, via telephone, or even using writings or web-based life in our cutting edge world, can start guidelines of our body and brain. Connections can inspire the soul of fun-loving nature and inventiveness or can loosen up us into a confiding in bond into another. Maybe you take part in a happy messaging trade with a companion. If you are in nearness with another, you can attempt relationship master, David Snarch's necessary, yet fantastic activity called "embracing until loose." The directions are to "take care of yourself, place your arms around your accomplice, centre around yourself, and to calm yourself down, the path down."

Inflammatory reactions assume a focal job in the improvement and diligence of numerous illnesses and can prompt weakening eternal agony. As a rule, irritation is your body's reaction to stretch. In this manner, lessening "battle or-flight" reactions in the sensory system and bringing down natural markers for stress can likewise decrease aggravation.

Ordinarily, specialists recommend prescriptions to battle aggravation. In any case, there's developing proof that another method to battle aggravation is by drawing in the vagus nerve and improving "vagal tone." This can be accomplished through day by day propensities, for example, yoga and contemplation—or in progressively extraordinary instances of irritation, for example, rheumatoid joint pain (RA)— by utilising an embedded gadget for vagus nerve incitement (VNS).

The vagus nerve is known as the "meandering nerve" since it has various branches that veer from two thick stems established in the cerebellum and brainstem that meander to the least viscera of your stomach area contacting your heart and most significant organs en route. Vagus signifies "meandering" in Latin. The words drifter, obscure, and vagrant are altogether gotten from a similar Latin root.

The vagus nerve is one of 12 sets of cranial nerves that start in the cerebrum and is a piece of the autonomic sensory system, which controls automatic body capacities. The nerve goes through the neck as it goes between the chest and midriff, and the lower some portion of the mind. It is associated with the engine works in the voice box, stomach, stomach, and heart and physical capacities in the ears and tongue. It is related to both driver and actual sizes in the sinuses and throat.

Vagus nerve incitement (VNS) sends standard, gentle beats of electrical vitality to the cerebrum using the vagus nerve, through a gadget that is like a pacemaker. There is no real inclusion of the cerebrum in this medical procedure, and patients can't by and large feel the beats. It is essential to remember that VNS is a treatment alternative restricted to choose people with epilepsy or treatment-safe sadness.

People with any of the accompanying criteria may conceivably be an inadmissible contender for VNS:

- One vagus nerve
- Accepting other simultaneous types of mind incitement
- Heart arrhythmias or different heart variations from the norm
- Dysautonomias (irregular working of the autonomic sensory system)
- Lung maladies or clutters (brevity of breath, asthma, and so on.)
- Ulcers (gastric, duodenal, and so on.)
- Vasovagal syncope (blacking out)
- Prior roughness
- VNS Implantation

This strategy, performed by a neurosurgeon, as a rule, takes around 45-an hour and a half with the patient most ordinarily under general anaesthesia. It usually works on an outpatient premise. Likewise, with all medical procedures, there is little danger of disease. Other careful risks of VNS incorporate irritation or torment at the entry point site, harm to close by nerves, and nerve narrowing.

Side impacts are most generally identified with incitement and, more often than not, improve after some time. These may incorporate any of the accompanyings:

- Roughness
- Expanded hacking
- Changes in voice/discourse
- General torment
- Throat or neck torment
- Throat or larynx fits
- Cerebral pain
- A sleeping disorder
- Acid reflux
- Muscle developments or jerking identified with the incitement
- Sickness or regurgitating

- The disabled feeling of touch
- Prickling or shivering of the skin

Of these, raspiness, hacking, throat tickling, and brevity of breath are the most well-known and are typically brief.

Patient Tips/Guidelines

If you have gotten VNS, you should screen your condition and generally speaking wellbeing intently. In the happen that any of the accompanyings happen, summon your primary care physician right:

- Continually dry voice
- Incitement which ends up difficult or sporadic
- Provocation which causes stifling, breathing or gulping troubles or an adjustment in pulse
- Changes in your degree of awareness, for example, expanded tiredness
- Signs that the beat generator may not be stimulating appropriately or that the battery is exhausted (the gadget quits working)
- Any new or irregular changes related explicitly to the incitement

What's more, you should call your doctor before you experience any medical tests that may influence, or be influenced by VNS, for example, attractive reverberation imaging (MRI), or before you have some other therapeutic gadgets embedded.

Chapter 10 Stimulation Of The Vagus Nerve And Keeping It Healthy

Keeping It Healthy

Since the vagus nerve plays such a critical role in our body, it is important to keep it healthy and do our best to avoid diseases that will alter the normal physiological processes of the nerve and create detrimental effects in our bodies. While there are many traditional medical and surgical ways that can positively impact the vagus nerve, our focus here will be more natural remedies. Something that has not received the attention it deserves. If we can help something naturally, without invasive surgery or medicines, then it is certainly worth looking into. The way we keep the vagus nerve healthy is by stimulating it. Stimulating the vagus nerve helps to strengthen the vagal tone. In turn, this effectively increases its ability to impact the body and activate the full use of it. We mentioned a variety of illnesses that can result from an unhealthy vagus nerve. It is important, then, to take the time necessary to make sure our own vagus nerve is not unhealthy. We are here to show you how.

Stimulation Of The Vagus Nerve

This is the crux of what we are here to talk about today: stimulating and activating the vagus nerve to reach its full potential. We have described just how crucial the vagus nerve is in our bodies. We detailed how many of the organ systems it has an impact on and what can occur if it does not function properly. Without a properly functioning vagus nerve, we are essentially doomed to nonstop illness and much worse. We are doomed to live a life where we will suffer tremendously due to depressed body systems. Does this sound too dramatic? Well, we are not speaking hyperbolically here. When we stimulate the vagus nerve, we strengthen it and unleash its full potential. There are numerous natural ways to stimulate the vagus nerve that will lead to tremendous health benefits down the line. Many of the natural ways to stimulate the vagus nerve are things that we do on a regular basis anyway. It will not be difficult to incorporate them into our lives and create countless health benefits for us. From laughing to deep breathing, we will describe what we can all do on a regular basis to stimulate the vagus nerve and keep it healthy.

The more conventional approaches for stimulation of the vagus nerve have been surgically implanted devices under the skin that feed wires directly to the vagus nerve. These wires send electrical impulses through the vagus nerve up to the brain. This direct stimulation is certainly the most effective and researched way of using simulation, which has been done extensively to help with epilepsy. The device is similar to an implanted defibrillator for the heart. The left vagus nerve is the common one used for this as the right vagus nerve is more likely to feed fibers directly to the heart. The risk, therefore, is much higher when trying to stimulate the right vagus nerve directly. Remember that each cranial nerve comes in a pair. According to the Mayo Clinic, the Food and Drug Administration has also approved the use of a noninvasive stimulation device to help stimulate the vagus nerve. This is a device that sits on top of the skin and provides stimulation through electrical impulses through the body and reaches the vagus nerve in a similar manner as the implanted device. The stimulation just won't be direct, but it will be effective.

These conventional methods are extremely beneficial, and multiple studies have shown their benefits in helping with seizures, headaches, depression, Post-traumatic stress disorder, anxiety, pain, and other illnesses. What we will focus on here are natural ways to stimulate the vagus nerve in order to have the same effects. While we are not suggesting that the techniques we discuss here will surpass or equal the results of the devices we just went over, we are suggesting that they will be beneficial and more convenient. Over time, they will strengthen the vagal tone and continue to activate the vagus nerve. All of these approaches can be done at home, and many of them can be done while performing our activities of daily living. If these practices work properly, it can save us from going through more invasive procedures. One thing to remember is that the only way to directly stimulate the vagus nerve is through some type of implanted device. The methods we discuss here are indirect but will still have favorable effects. Let's begin dissecting some of them now.

The vagus nerve innervates several portions of the body as it runs along its pathway after leaving the brainstem. It is by far the most crucial of the crucial nerves. This definitely means a lot. Doing specific exercises that will target these specific areas is critical in stimulating the vagus nerve. This means that where the vagus nerve goes, are the areas we must target. Perform these simple techniques, and you will be amazed at what can occur. You may not feel radical effects right off the bat. The purpose of these techniques is to provide small amounts of improvement with each one that will create a more far-reaching effect down the line. With each exercise, we are strengthening the vagal tone, and as a result, creating a healthier vagus nerve. One of the criteria for performing the following techniques is to be consistent and do them regularly. They are not a one and done miracle cure. They are to be incorporated into a healthy overall lifestyle. Nothing good comes easy. Just like when we are trying to get abs, we must consistently target these muscles with specific exercises and routines. We must do these exercises on a regular basis in order for them to have the results we want. We must invest a lot of time and energy. It's okay though, because the investment is for our health. Our health is always worth our time. You may not have realized how beneficial these tasks could be, but you were probably already doing many of them. Now, we have finally arrived at the main portion of this book. We will learn how to naturally access, activate and stimulate the vagus nerve and improve our own ability to heal ourselves.

Humming

That's right, just like the birds, we must hum and be at peace. Have you ever seen a stressed-out hummingbird? I don't think we have. Perhaps we should ask, though.

The vagus nerve passes through the facial area close to our vocal cords and inner ear. The vibrations from the humming that we perform can help to stimulate the vagus nerve and significantly influence the nervous system and other parts of the body. This is probably the most effective way to target this particular portion of the vagus nerve. It is best to find a quiet area where you can hum in peace without so many distractions. A quiet room or an open and empty field will suffice. A common activity where people perform humming is yoga. Taking a yoga class can be tremendously beneficial for vagus nerve health. Another activity is meditation. Try learning these activities and see where they take you. We will get more in-depth with these two activities later. Humming may be one of the simplest exercises to perform. Do it on a regular basis, and you will experience positive results.

To hum properly, we must create a low continuous vibrating sound. It is basically like singing with our lips closed and allowing the sound to travel out through the nose. The humming must be smooth and prolonged, rather than rapid and erratic. The continuous smooth vibration is what ultimately targets the vagus nerve in the facial area. Literally, we can do this exercise anywhere and at any time. Try it out several times a day and see how it feels. If you do it properly, you can actually feel the vibrations along the side of your face and ear.

Deep Breathing Exercises

We breathe every moment of the day, right? So, we can just skip this . Well, not exactly. This is a particular type of breathing we are talking about here. Conscious deep breathing is another great exercise to help stimulate the vagus nerve naturally. The reason we say conscious is that they are breaths we must think about and do appropriately. Of course, all of us breathe every moment of every day. Even when we are sleeping, we are breathing. We know this because we are able to wake up the next day. These breaths are sufficient to sustain life, but not enough to stimulate the vagus nerve in any way. The way to do this properly is to take deep breaths in an appropriate way to target specific body parts that will activate the vagus nerve. The aim of these breaths is to move the belly and diaphragm and slow down your breathing tremendously. The movement of the abdominal muscles in this manner will help to specifically target the portion of the vagus nerve that innervates the organs in this cavity. Remember that the vagus nerve ends in the abdominal cavity. We must contract our abdominal muscles deep inwards in order to effectively reach the vagus nerve.

On a regular basis, when we are just walking around, the number of breaths we take is anywhere from 12-20 per minute. This will certainly be increased when we are more active, like running or hiking. When we are performing conscious deep breathing, we must slow these breaths down to about five to seven per minute so that each breath is efficient. When we take a breath, we should spend at least three to five seconds inhaling, then holding our breath for about three seconds, and then take five to 10 seconds exhaling. When we take these extended breaths, we must take aim to move our belly and diaphragm in and out. Taking slow breaths and holding them for several seconds will allow us to exercise the vagus nerve as we target the specific organs that will stimulate the vagus nerve. We cannot cheat here. We have to do this with every breath in order to get the full effect. If you can do this about five to 10 times throughout the day, it is perfect. If you couple it with the other practices on this list, it will be even more beneficial.

You can do deep breathing exercises several times a day while doing your regular activities. Some of the most appropriate times are when you are watching TV, lying in bed, washing dishes, sitting at a computer, or even driving your car. Conscious deep breathing is a great exercise to perform that will not interrupt your day. Make sure you find a place where you are alone because people love to interrupt. Especially when they don't know what is going on. Take full advantage of this. Deep breathing will target the most major parts of the vagus nerve as it will involve the abdomen and thorax, where the most critical organs run through.

Notice how, after doing an intense exercise that people are breathing rapidly. Of course, they are doing this to help increase the intake of oxygen that the muscles demand. Not only is the breathing rapid, but the heart rate also increases immensely to meet the demands of the body. The body is basically on overdrive at this point, and the sympathetic nervous system is in full swing. One thing people will do to help themselves recover is to slow everything down. When they stand straight up and begin taking slow deep breaths, this will effectively target the vagus nerve and reduce the heart rate, putting the body in a state of rest. This will work pretty much every time. If you are feeling out of control and can't seem to settle down, try taking some deep breaths. This will relax your body and physiological process and allow you to work and think more efficiently. Conscious deep breathing can help us in many ways, and many of us were probably doing them anyway. Out of all of the techniques we discuss in this , this one may be one of the simplest and most effective, so definitely take the time to try them out.

The Valsalva Maneuver

The name may sound complicated, but the technique really isn't. It is performed by basically trying to exhale against a closed airway. Close your mouth and pinch your nose, then exhale. You may feel your ears pop. You have probably done this multiple times while driving in a car or flying in an airplane when your ears felt like they were stuffed. Well, when you were doing this exercise, you were doing something more beneficial than you even realized. Performing the Valsalva maneuver increases the pressure in your chest cavity, which increases your vagal tone and effectively helps to stimulate the vagus nerve. This particular maneuver has been performed multiple times to help a person reduce their heart rate. There was a situation on a major airline flight a few years back where a passenger began having rapid heart rates into the 120s and 130s. They were feeling dizzy and faint and noticed the palpitations in their chests. They tried to ignore the situation but eventually had to reach out for help. Luckily, there was a seasoned medical professional on board, and they told this person to basically perform the Valsalva maneuver several times for several seconds. Within a couple of minutes, the heart rate was back down into the 80s and 90s. Once this occurred, they had the passenger take some deep breaths and use some supplemental oxygen that was onboard. Of course, the person received a further medical evaluation as a precaution after they landed; however, for the moment, this maneuver may have saved the person's life. The Valsalva Maneuver has been used for years to help reduce and normalize the heart rate. Now we know it is all because we are targeting the vagus nerve.

This was definitely an extreme example, and we hope that it never comes to this for you. However, this situation truly illustrates the efficacy of the Valsalva Maneuver. Try it a couple of times a day in conjunction with other techniques we have and see where it takes you. This is another exercise you can do just about anywhere, and it literally takes a few seconds. Make sure not to overstrain and go beyond your comfort level, or other problems may occur.

Cold Exposure

Many prominent people, including several athletes and high-profile celebrities, have promoted the idea of cold exposure. They have credited it with helping them start their day with a bang and making them more productive. The increase in vagal tone helped them feel more energized and attentive. There is a reason for that. Many people think you would actually be more energized with the sympathetic response. When in reality, it wears you down more due to the excessive use of energy. When the parasympathetic response kicks in and everything is calm and loosened up, is when energy storage really occurs. Since cold exposure will activate the parasympathetic response, it will increase our energy and productivity.

We admit this may be the least appealing technique to stimulate the vagus nerve we have so far. However, if the results are real, then regular, or at least occasional, cold exposure may be worth it in the end. Many researchers have found that regular cold exposure can inhibit the sympathetic response and really elevate the parasympathetic response via the vagus nerve. Many people will take cold showers or go out into the cool air with minimal clothing. We are not saying you have to walk around in freezing cold weather in a bathing suit. That may be too extreme. However, making yourself a little uncomfortable by exposing yourself to the cold may have tremendous benefits for your overall health. Sometimes to make positive changes, we have to put ourselves in uncomfortable positions.

A good way to do this is to ease into it and take it slowly. Certainly, if you jump into an extreme element without taking the proper care, it can create other problems as well. We certainly don't want you to do that. The best thing to do is to take it step by step. Instead of just walking out in freezing cold weather the first-day wearing shorts and flip flops, perhaps you can try immersing just your face into cold water for a tolerable amount of time. Maybe go outside with one less covering than you're used to. After that, just work up the ladder. Stand in a tub with just your feet immersed in cold water and then work up from there until you are able to take cold showers regularly. Taking small progressive steps on a daily basis is the way to go. Overall, cold exposure has been shown to activate the vagus nerve and also the neurons in the vagus nerve pathway. Once again, this may the hardest one to talk you into, but the results will be worth it. Try it out and see where it takes you.

Exercise

Exercise has been shown to significantly affect and stimulate the vagus nerve and support overall brain health as well. Exercises that can target the core abdominal muscles are especially useful. Exercise also improves your conditioning and significantly increases your energy. Find physical activities you love doing and get moving. A good exercise session can also release certain naturally occurring hormones that will enhance the vagus nerve response via the parasympathetic nervous system. Follow this up with some deep breathing exercises, and you are gold.

Massage

Who doesn't love a good massage session? Honestly, we think everyone does. Getting regular massages has been shown to help to stimulate vagus nerve activity. Specifically, massaging certain areas of the body like the feet and the carotid sinus on the side of the neck has been shown to decrease the sympathetic response and stimulate the vagus nerve, effectively increasing the parasympathetic response. Some research has even shown that massaging the carotid sinus can help to decrease seizures. Massaging the abdomen and getting deep into the tissues has been known to have a positive response in stimulating the vagus nerve as well. It is recommended to get these massages done by a professional in the field as they can be intricate and precise and also cause severe injury if not done correctly.

These specific massages do not have to be done on a daily basis. If you can get them done a couple of times a month, coupled with the other practices in this , that should be sufficient. A good massage by a well-trained therapist will not only make you feel good, but it will also be good for you. The key is to make sure they target the areas we . A back massage may feel good, but may not do much good in targeting the vagus nerve.

Having A Good Time

What are we talking about here? Yes, laughing and socializing with friends is known to improve vagal tone and stimulate the vagus nerve. So, if you're putting off some work, you need to do to spend time with friends, don't feel too guilty. A healthy amount of socialization is needed in our lives. We are not saying you have to party and drink every single day. However, a healthy balance of socializing is extremely important in stimulating the vagus never and improving overall health. All work and no play just won't cut it. Laughing and smiling regularly has been shown to target and stimulate certain areas of the vagus nerve in the face. So, do this that makes you smile more. As well, just smile for no reason. People will wonder what you are up to. Just like with exercise, laughing and genuinely being happy releases certain hormones in the body that will positively target the vagus nerve. We will discuss the endocrine system, which produces these varying hormones later on in this book.

Yoga

Yes, yoga can be positively impactful for the vagus nerve. Many of the techniques we have already mentioned, like deep breathing, are a part of a good yoga workout. Plus, yoga itself involves many stretches, poses, and positions that target the vagus nerve, and help stimulate it so it can perform at maximum capacity. Yoga is pretty easy to learn for the simple fact that we can find yoga studios on just about any street corner nowadays. It is advised you learn from a professional at least the first couple of times before doing it on your own. When you are knowledgeable, then yoga training can be performed just about anywhere.

Chapter 11 Vagus Nerve For Reducing Inflammation

Linkage Between Stress, Inflammation And The Immune System

The vagus nerve (Crane Nerve X) is the main nerve of the autonomous nervous system's parasympathetic division (rest and digestion). It is an essential way of communication between the heart, cardiovascular system, digestive system and immune system. This bi-directional nervous path passes through the chest and abdomen and is connected to several organs.

The body is closely linked and the Vagus nerve plays a major role in organizing interaction. Signals from the brain are conveyed to the chest and abdominal organ and back to the central nervous system from the intestines and lungs. The Vagus nerve helps to create this communication network by signalling the brain to produce neurotransmitters and hormones, to organize reactions, to regulate stress reactions and to keep inflammation under control.

In controlling the parasympathetic rest, for instance, the vagus nerve plays a central role in helping to regulate breathing and heart rate, promote relaxation, stimulate digestion and create a sense of peace and calmness. The Vagus nerve releases neurotransmitters acetylcholine to help coordinate this calming reaction, which tends to be a significant brake on inflammation in the corpse.

Vagal Tone And Its Benefits

Since it is a major control center for the body, this nerve's health is of utmost importance to your brain, your immune system and your overall inflammatory condition.

Many individuals have more vagus nerve function than others, allowing their bodies to relax after stress more quickly. Your Vagus response's intensity is known as vagal tone.

Low vagal tone with chronic inflammation was associated. Research shows that the cardiac amplitude, an indicator of reduced vagal tone, is often decreased in inflammatory conditions such as arthritis and other autoimmune diseases. This decreased vagal tone allows proinflammable cytokines (inflammatory substances that damage other cells and tissues) to become more active, leading to systemic inflammation, which leads to greater sympathetic nervous system activity and stress hormones.

Abdominal Massage As A Natural Anti- Inflammatory

Luckily, this nerve can be activated and your vagal tone improved by natural therapies, which help balance your immune system, relaxed body and mind, and lower inflammation. Research demonstrates that the Vagus nerve stimulation acts as a natural anti-inflammatory and calming agent, as it decreases the development of pro-inflammatory cytokines and calms the nervous system.

A method of self-abdominal massage is an evolving technique for reducing inflammation and tone of the vagus nerve. Gentle pressure massage has been shown to stimulate the vagus nervous system, increase digestive movements and content, and boost insulin secretion in pre-term infants to regulate their blood sugar (adult trials are still required). The combination of manual handling and stimulation of the Vagus nerve can have strong anti-inflammatory advantages.

How to Carry out Abdominal Massage

This abdominal massage technique is simple to do at home in just a few minutes. This procedure is best performed on an empty stomach a few hours after eating. Start slowly and see the reactions of your body.

1. Lie on a soft floor mat or on a mattress.

2. Place your hand under your breastbone or sternum. Make gentle motions downward — drive your hand down to the abdomen. Do this step a few minutes, cycle one hand over the other in a reverse motion like bicycle pedaling.

3. First, make small circular motions on your abdomen with your fingertips. Begin to massage the sides of your abdomen and slowly move back and forth. Go deeper and deeper with a strong yet relaxed pressure. For a few minutes, start this abdominal massage.

4. Finish your practice with a gentle, reclining two-knee spinal twist (Supta Matsyendrasana) for some minutes. The restorative yoga pose increases the digestion and encourages an opening of the fascia and diaphragm to help you deepen your breath.

- Lying on your back, exhale softly into a floor or mattress as you press your lower back.

- Breathe a few moments here as you open your lower back.

- When ready, gently relax the abdominal muscles and bend your knees to the chest.

- Breathe out , then lower your arms to the floor, even with your back, with your hands at your side.

- As you inhale slowly, raise your feet a little higher than your knees and slowly exhale both legs toward the floor toward the left.

- Keep your knees and your feet and knees lined together at the bottom of your hips. Remain 30 to 60 seconds in this position.

- Begin to breathe deeply and steadily, as you softly move with your breath from side to side.

Try this simple practice for your Vagus nerve power. Carryout the following exercises once or twice a day for several weeks for a few minutes. The benefits of lower pressure, enhanced digestion, better detoxification, reduced pain and squelched inflammation can surprise you!

Vagus Nerve Stimulation (Vns) For Depression And Flow State

Vagus nerve stimulation has been proven to help most people to overcome feelings of anxiety and flow state. I am so passionate about this field of work because it can be the key to opening the door to a newly found liberation for those who struggle on a physical, mental and emotional basis.

It's all about how we think at an emotional level, how we interact with others and how successful we can be. It also has a crucial impact on our physical health.

The vagus nerve stretches from the brain stem to the lower abdomen's viscera and touches almost all organs. This is related to the autonomous nervous system: an unconscious mechanism that is unintended.

The "ZONE" you are in affects a great deal on the filter you use to experience the world. Whether you feel anxious or comfortable, if your body is tense or relaxed, if your mind is thinking or calm, and if you are able to think clearly, how things taste, smell and sound.

Neuroception refers to the way we test for danger. Our nervous system talks if you encounter someone, something like; are you safe or are you dangerous? If we have a deadline, our nervous system will check for our danger to our safety.

Neuroception is automatic and rapid and will be affected by the fitness and variation of our Vagus Nerve. In how we see the world and have three regions, our autonomic state is the most important thing.

Green zone is our safe zone, where every other social engagements can take place.

- Heart rate slows down
- Stimulation of saliva and digestion
- Activation of facial muscles for connection
- Improved vocal and eye contact for connection
- Muscles in the center of the ear turn on to raise the mid-range volume to hear others' voices.
- Essentially in this zone, our sense of sight, smell, sound, and vision change so that we are prepared for digestion and engagement.

The Yellow Zone is the state of danger: Fight-and-Flight: do I run or fight, like hell?

- Heart rate increases
- Flat and smooth facial effect

- Auditory system changes: muscles in the center of the ear shift to help distinguish low frequency noises and high frequency sounds for attackers.

- Pupils dilate

- Blood moves away from the digestive system.

The Red Zone is the Life-threatening zone (The Freeze Zone)

This is the peak where the nervous system feels they will die and immobilization takes place. It's known as death pretenders and it is the reptilian response that needs to be seen with this eye, the oldest part of our brain and injury. It is not to run but to freeze the one common response to traumatic events. We are disassociated or shut down and this is entirely unintentional.

Healthy people can easily switch between the green and the yellow system, which is why the vagus nerve is so significant. It is a challenge to know whether there is security or danger and to send that message to every organ in the body so that they are able to answer in kind.

80 percent of your Vagus nerve fibers descend to your organs and say safety or danger and 20 percent reassert safety or danger to reinstate the data.

The Vagus Nerve functions as a neural brake-so that the body slows down when it acts in the green zone.

The Vagus nerve has a second branch that functions as a buffer, but is connected to life-threatening incidents. In comparison to the green region that slows you to relax, it slows you to dissociate, causing people to freeze or dissociate themselves and what is turned on in traumatic situations. It's like the freezes reptile.

After a traumatic event, many people ask: why did I freeze? Because your nervous system chose to die and you had no control.

Why does it all look, smell and taste different? Because it is linked to any device in your body based on what you've done.

Why am I still worried? Anxiety is an overactive mechanism of neuroception where the body interprets threats where no threat is present. And we're wired like that. We have a NERVOUS system-we are negatively influenced by risk and need it to survive. We are searching for danger.

In the olden days, we referred to danger by lions chasing us. Today, it means missing a deadline or some sorts of appointments, but these same neural pathways are activated and you feel frightened.

Even in non-frightening cases, our body responds to the same neutral pathways, such as missing a train or that are late for an appointment or traffic, our body is on the same neural pathways that once have been reserved for "I don't have enough food to survive," and you always feel like crap.

The body tends to overestimate the risk of this' nerve' process.

Why does trauma last so long and why is it so hard to treat? Trauma is physiological, not psychological. Trauma is a sort of rearrangement of how the whole body works. It is not enough just to view it as a question of feeling bad and getting something to conquer. And this is the case for a lot of issues, such as anxiety, borderline personality disorder.

Low Vagal Tone

Feeling safe and in the green zone is crucial.

- This takes us to the flow state to enhance critical thinking, productivity, and learning.

- This activates healthy and beneficial hormones

- Makes life easier and more enjoyable.

- Allows the movement of the body. Most people with trauma are suffering from IBS. This doesn't make no sense from a logical point of view, but from the nervous system we see that all these are connected by the vagus nerve together. Good health is fully associated with the vagus nerve.

- This makes people like you because, thanks to mirror neurons, we are prepared for connection in the green zone.

- It optimizes the entire human experience.

The condition in which we find ourselves mostly will impact our entire human experience: the way we feel within ourselves, our emotional responses, our ability to connect with the ones we love, our ability to work and develop.

Healthy people can easily switch between the green and yellow system and that is why the vagus nerve is so critical and why I think stimulation of the vagus nerve is necessary during long periods of stress. It's a challenge to tell whether protection or danger exists and give this message to every organ in the body in order to answer in the same way.

Vagus Nerve Stimulation (Vns) For Depression

This is surgical process that can be used in treating people with treatment-resistant depression. The implanted device like a pacemaker is connected to a relaxing wire which is threaded along the nerve called the vagus nerve. The vagus nerve passes up the neck to the brain, linking regions that are supposed to be part of the mood regulation. When implanted, this system provides the vagus nerve with daily electrical impulse.

How Vagus Nerve Stimulation Works

Once the VNS operation is completed, a little battery-powered device will be inserted into your neck-the size of a silver dollar. It acts as a pacemaker. Another incision is made at the left side of the neck, and a thin wire (located just below the skin) runs from the apparatus to the major vagus nerve. The machine sends electric pulses into the nerve, transmitting them into the brain.

Such electrical pulses transmitted via the vagus nerve to the brain may alleviate the symptoms of depression for reasons that doctors do not fully comprehend. Impulse can influence how nerve cell circuits transmit signals in mood-affecting parts of the brain. However, it takes a few months before you feel the effects, though.

If applicable, the system settings (essentially dose change) in the office with a programming wall can be changed by the doctor. The system is usually set to go off periodically. You can also disable it with a special magnet.

Research on the effect of VNS on people with clinical depression has been generally positive. A research in 2005 compared 124 people who were receiving usual treatment with 205 people who received usual treatment plus VNS. Biological psychiatryin The hybrid treatment group showed more progress than the normal treatment group after one year of treatment. Among 27% of patients who received VNS, there was a significant improvement compared to 13% who did not. VNS is not fast anxiety treatment. Studies show that a treatment response can take up to 9 months on average.

VNS Risks and Side Effects

This include, cough, brief hoarseness, or shortness of breath may have side effects of the VNS. Most of these side effects arise in the 30 seconds on which the stimulator is triggered. The implantation process, like any operation, poses some risks of infection. Unlike pacemakers, when it is used out, you will finally require surgery to replace the plug. Additionally, while uncommon, system or lead damage may require additional surgery before the battery is replaced.

As the VNS system may interfere with mammograms, special positioning may be necessary to obtain the best possible image. Other medical procedures, such as heart defibrillation and ultrasound, may also affect the VNS system. Therefore, special precautions may be required before an MRI scan, so make sure your doctor knows.

You will probably continue other therapies for your anxiety, such as depression and counseling, even when you are treated with VNS.

Vagus Nerve Stimulation Therapy For Ptsd

Researchers at the University of Dallas, Texas are studying how moderate vagus nerve stimulation can help alleviate the symptoms of post-traumatic stress disorder (PTSD).

The vagus nerve regulates the sympathetic nervous system which tracks a vast range of essential bodily functions, including digestion and heart rate slowing.

Vagus nerve stimulation (VNS) has been shown to enhance memory retention as a treatment for conditions including epilepsy and depression.

The effect of the technique on memory is essential: UT Dallas researchers theorized that it could help people with PTSD effectively resolve the fear response in circumstances that are not threatened.

UT Dallas scientists found that moderate electrical pulses to the vagus nerve also had some effects on defense against PTSD symptoms in a recent preclinical study published in the journal Translational Psychiatry.

"We found evidence that a treatment for traumatic memory has brought significant changes to other symptoms of PTSD, such as anxiety, agitation and avoidance," Dr Christa McIntyre, Associate Professor of Neuroscience at the Brain and Behavioral University, and the senior author of the study, said.

In mice with PTSD symptoms, scientists applied painless electric stimulation to the vagus nerve. Such signs included responses to fear and anxiety in conditions without risks and reduced social experiences.

After VNS, there were reduced responses to fear and social interaction in animals, indicating that therapy was effective in reducing symptoms of PTSD. When VNS is the same advantage to humans, the latest treatments can be effective supplementary, said Dr. Michael Kilgard, neuroscience professor at UT Dallas, and study writer.

"Such therapies commonly in use for PTSD patients include speech therapy and exposure therapy, which can help, but understandably patients do not always pursue such interventions as they do not want to undergo more trauma," said Margaret Fonde Jonsson Professor, Kilgard. "We wanted to explore ways to improve sensitivity and effectiveness of the therapy." Kilgard explained that changes for people with PTSD may not be long-lasting though they are faithful to current treatments. If you encounter a new tragedy in your life, for instance, death in the family, you usually lose a lot of your gains instead of having mild declines in PTSD symptoms.

"In our study, we found that VNS not only strengthened the reaction of fear in non-stressful situations, but also persisted after another traumatic experience," said Kilgard.

Researchers also found that VNS therapy provided protection after full discontinuation of treatment.

"We were excited to discover that there were protective effects after one week of no VNS therapy at all," said Lindsey Noble, lead author and doctoral student at UT Dallas. "We really want to know more about this and see if VNS can provide more benefits for other conditions, such as obsessive compulsive disorders and dependence across the board."

Vagus Nerve Stimulation Therapy For Addiction

VNS therapy may help addicts in overcoming substance abuse, according to an effective preclinical review, which is the extinction of conditioned drug-seeking behaviors.

In the January issue of Learning and Memory, the new report "Vagus Nerve Stimulation Reduces cocaine quest and age plastics in the network extinction" has been released.

While this is an experimental study, researchers believe that their results can potentially be applied to people battling drug addiction and substance-abuse disorders. VNS treatment for certain disorders, including clinical depression, epilepsy and inflammation, has already been approved by the FDA.

The new research contributes to an increasing number of data on the advantages of VNS therapy. For example, February 2016 study found that VNS therapy enhanced default mode network connectivity which decreased Major Depressive Disorders (MDD) symptoms.

Furthermore, a research by neuroscientists and immunologists conducted in July 2016 found that VNS therapy blocked the "inflammatory reflex" by blocking pro-inflammatory cytokines output. This research was the first human study to reduce rheumatoid arthritis symptoms by causing a chain reaction that reduces cytokine levels and inflammation.

Researchers at Dallas School of Behavioral and Brain Sciences at the University of Texas found, during the new January 2017 report, that lab rats who became cocaine users decreased their drug-seeking behavior dramatically when treated with VNS therapy.

Researchers found that VNS therapy has induced improvements in synaptic plasticity in cocaine-addicted laboratory rats between prefrontal cortex and amygdala. VNS seemed to promote the "extinction training" of drug-seeking habits by increasing cravings and encrypting new reward behaviors in place of former drug-induced lever-related ones to get a cocaine hit.

In Latin, vagus means "wandering". The vagus nerve is also referred to as the "wandering nerve," because it has many branches which are different from the cerebellum's thick stems (Latin for "small brain") and the brainstem that wanders to the lowest viscera of the abdomen, which are affecting your heart and most of your major organ. The vagus nerves are a central player in the "good brain axis." In 1921, a nobel laureate German physiologist, Otto Loewi, noticed that vagus stimulation decreased the heart rate by inducing the release of the substance he called Vagusstoff. The "vagus material," later identified by scientists as acetylcholine, was the first neurotransmitter ever to be detected.

Vagus substance (acetylcholine) is like a tranquilizer which can be offered easily by taking quick, slow diaphragm breaths. Tapping your vagus nerve's energy actively could lead to inner relaxation while reducing stress and taming your inflammatory reflex at a neurobiologic stage.

The vagus nerve is the primary component of the parasympathetic nervous system which controls the response of "rest and digest" and "tend and mate." On the reverse side, the sympathetic nervous system encourages "fight or flight" response to preserve homeostasis.

A slight increase in heart rate as you inhale and a drop in the heart rate as you exhale are the natural indications for a healthy vagal tone. A higher vagal tone index is associated with positive emotions and psychological balance, which triggers an upward spiral of well-being. In addition, a low vagal tone index is associated with floating anxiety, stress, inflammation, and depression that can lead to a declining spiral of well-being.

Vagus Nerve Stimulation Can Decrease Drug Addictions via Synaptic Plasticity

The latest research on VNS therapy shows the potential to decrease drug addictions by enhancing the functional connection between Prefrontal Cortex (PFC) and Basi-Lateral Amygdala (BLA) by stimulating the vagus nerve with a mild electric current. Immunohistochemistry has been used by researchers to track changes in the PFC and BLA, which function to control cue learning and extinction.

Drug and alcohol abuse disorders typically cause PFC and other brain regions changes that affect the inhibitory regulation of drug-seeker behavior. To eradicate hardwired addictive behavior patterns, researchers at UT Dallas found that it is necessary to break the paired relationship between drug-associated indices and pay for extinction which fuels dependence during a learning phase.

Senior author of this research Sven Kroener summarized his team's results in a declaration at the University of Texas in Dallas today: "We are researching extinction training and how vagus nerve stimulation may help subjects develop a New Behavior which opposes a current, maladaptive behavior like narcotics. However, the extinction of drug-seeking memories and extinction of fearful memories rely on the same pathway/Substrate In the brain. In our research, vagus nerve stimulation take into consideration the two extinction learning process and reduces the relapse as well."

This technique can really become a treatment during recovery, where people are doing these exposure treatments, looking at the triggers that caused their desire when abstaining from a safe situation. The VNS therapy can reinforce this abstinence and wean them away from drug-related activity and protect them from cravings.

You also research how distinctly activated nerves can help treat post-traumatic stress disorder (PTSD), depression, tinnitus, and help people recover from stroke paralysis. Perhaps their latest findings on the possible use of VNS therapy in human clinical trials will soon be.

Conclusion

Thank you for making it through to the end. In an ideal world, we would be free of ailments and disease, but in reality, our bodies are subject to external and internal threats that ultimately impact on our physical health and mental wellbeing. This is what necessitates the autonomic nervous system to trigger responses that are appropriate to the prevailing conditions in both the internal body environment and external surroundings.

Our greatest weapons against ill health and physical disorders ultimately lie in our understanding of how our body functions and in what way we can improve natural mechanisms to make it even more effective in self-renewal and repair. It is for this reason that we have gone through the Vagus nerve and its functions in the body as relates to good health.

By fully comprehending the healing potential that is contained in the vagus nerve, you have equipped yourself with the knowledge that will guide in taking a more natural approach to maintaining a healthy body. When we work together with our natural instincts and reflexes, we reap more in terms of creating the right homeostatic balance for body organs and processes to function.

Your understanding of the importance of vagal activity puts you in a unique position to change your outcomes and start living a healthier and happier life. We may not be able to avoid all illnesses and infections, but we can certainly reduce the frequency and severity of the disorders we routinely have to face.

The vagus nerve plays a crucial role in your overall health, and by taking the initiative to learn how it functions and how you can activate it, you have started your journey to unleashing your body's natural self-healing powers.

The next step is to start applying the techniques that you have learned in this book and following the guidelines provided consistently to achieve the best vagal tone possible, which will, in turn, translate into numerous health benefits for you.

www.ingramcontent.com/pod-product-compliance
Lightning Source LLC
Chambersburg PA
CBHW071403210526
45465CB00001B/224